"Knowing yourself is the
beginning of all wisdom"

—Aristotle

70 & ABOVE

GENETIC THREADS

NAVIGATING CONFIDENCE IN THE FABRIC OF LIFE

DR. M.K. SHINGARI

Research & Development Centre

Chromatography & Instruments Company, Vadodara

Editor

Edited by:

Mr. G.K. Vithal

Outstanding Scientist

Ex. GM (PC&AL), Heavy Water Board,

Department of Atomic Energy

Assisted By:

Ms. Nida Amiri, Mr. Arya Shingari and Mr. Ashok Patel

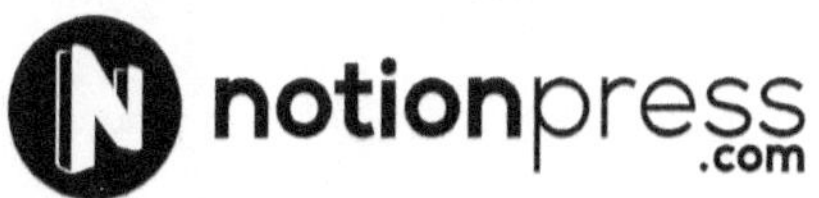

INDIA • SINGAPORE • MALAYSIA

ISBN
Paperback 979-8-89724-268-9
Hardcase 979-8-89744-283-6

Contents

Acknowledgments	7

About the Author	9

Foreword	13

Book Review	15

An Open Letter to Super Seniors	17

1. Introduction	21

2. Aging and it's Side Effects	25

3. Nature (Genes) vs Nurture
(Environmental Influences)	38

4. Positive Psychology and Aging
(Understanding the Influence
of Positive Psychology on Behaviour
and Well-Being in Seniors)	46

5. Mental Health and Well-Being in Old Age	57

6. Spirituality and Aging	63

7. Aging, Quality of Life, and
    Social Support Available   73

8. Medical Aspects: Cardiovascular Diseases,
    Strokes, Cancer & Other Age-Related Diseases   87

9. Real Life Examples   96

10. Aging Gracefully
    (Essential Health Strategies for Seniors)   114

11. Suggestions and Conclusion   127

Appnedix 1   The Secrets of Old Age   133

Appendix 2   Dangerous Age Group   137

Appendix 3   Yoga Exercises for Seniors   146

Appendix 4   DO's and DO NOT's for
              Seniors Aged 70 and Above   172

Appendix 5   Five Daily Habits to be adopted
              By Seniors around 70's   179

Acknowledgments

Mr. Girish Kumar Vithal is an Outstanding Scientist of Heavy Water Board, Department of Atomic Energy, Government of India and my very old family friend, who consider me more than his elder brother. I am profoundly grateful to him for his invaluable contributions to this book, Genetic Threads – Navigating Confidence in the Fabric of Life. His extraordinary efforts in editing this manuscript have been pivotal in shaping it into its final form. Despite numerous rounds of additions, deletions, and revisions, his unwavering commitment to refining the content has been truly inspiring. Mr. Vithal also provided exceptional guidance, engaging in detailed discussions on several technical issues and simplifying complex concepts to make them easily understandable, using simple language to the majority of readers of all levels.

I sincerely acknowledge the support of my Doctor friends and others who provided valuable Scientific inputs to validate my experiences.

I extend my heartfelt gratitude to Shri Ashok Kumar Patel for his meticulous efforts in transcribing my dictations and assisting with the typing of the manuscript. His dedication and patience have been instrumental in ensuring the smooth progress of this work.

I would also like to acknowledge Ms. Nida Amiri for her assistance in sourcing information through Google and providing valuable inputs that enriched the content of this book. Her contributions have added depth and precision to the narrative.

A special note of thanks goes to my wife, Dr. (Mrs.) Kiran Shingari, and my sons, Gaurav, Amar and their families for their unconditional support and encouragement throughout this journey. Their understanding, patience, and unwavering belief in me made it possible to complete this book within the remarkably short span of three months.

Finally, to all who have directly or indirectly supported me in this endeavor, I express my sincere appreciation and gratitude.

—Dr. M.K. Shingari

Author

About the Author

Dr. Mahender Kumar Shingari, Ph.D. in Chemical Engineering from the United Kingdom, is a vibrant and **principled individual, even at the age of 85.** I have had the privilege of knowing him since 1982 and I can confidently say he is an **inspiring personality.** Born to refugee parents, Dr. Shingari started life with nothing but a vision for higher education and excellence. His perseverance led him to establish the Chromatography Instrument Company in Vadodara, which has significantly contributed to Indian industries by developing indigenous scientific products.

His Recent Publication **'Ek Refugee Scientist' Author's Autobiography,** launched by Himachal Pradesh Chief Minister, Shri Sukhvinder Singh Sukhu, on 24th July, 2024 was extensively covered by the Media. Comments from 'The Tribune', Chandigarh:

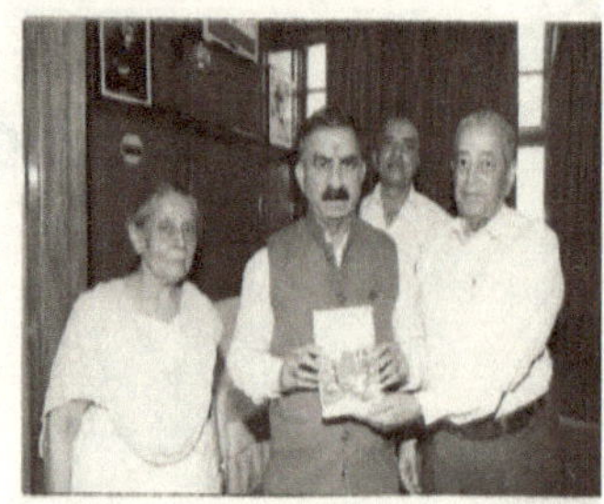

Sukhu releases *Ek Refugee Scientist*

SHIMLA, JULY 24

Chief Minister Sukhvinder Singh Sukhu here today released *Ek Refugee Scientist*, an autobiography penned by Dr MK Shingari of Solan district.

He lauded Dr Shingari's work and extended his best wishes for the success of the new publication.

The CM said the book would serve as an inspiration for the younger generation. This autobiography marks Dr Shingari's fifth book. — TNS

CM Sukhu at the book release on Wednesday. TRIBUNE PHOTO

The book beautifully captures his Extraordinary journey of his rise from humble beginnings to becoming a successful Industrialist. It is available on Indian e-commerce platforms such as Amazon.in, Flipkart, and the Notion Press Store, as well as globally on Amazon.com, Amazon.ca, and Amazon.co.uk . Digital editions can also be accessed on platforms like Kindle, iBooks, Google Books, and Kobo, ensuring his inspiring story reaches readers worldwide.

This serves as a testament to his dedication, hard work, and commitment to excellence. Dr. Shingari remains a grounded and humble individual who never forgets his past and has instilled these values in his family.

Apart from his professional achievements, Dr. Shingari is a true friend, a nature lover, and always ready to support his friends and employees. His magnetic personality at 85 can be attributed to his disciplined lifestyle.

Daily Routine and Lifestyle

Dr. Shingari's day begins at 3:00 AM with a glass of warm water and his morning medicine. He then engages in light exercises and a morning walk. Around 6:30 AM, he consumes three glasses of water mixed with Amla and Aloe Vera juice, followed by a nutritious breakfast of mixed dry fruits, milk with turmeric, bread, and eggs or sometimes a traditional sweet, *pinni*.

By 9:00 AM, Dr. Shingari is at his company, meeting employees and approving documents until 2:00 PM. He returns home for a light lunch consisting of one *roti*, vegetables, half a glass of buttermilk, and occasionally a small dessert like *gajar ka halwa* or *ghajak*.

In the evening, he enjoys a cup of soup or light snacks before a small dinner around 7:00 PM, which may include an item like *idli* or *dosa*. He retires to bed by 7:30 PM, adhering to this routine with remarkable consistency. Despite facing age-related health challenges, he maintains a positive attitude and takes his medicines promptly.

The Inspiration Behind This Book

As a friend, philosopher, and guide, Dr. Shingari has inspired countless individuals, including me. I persuaded him to pen down his life experiences and advice in a document that would benefit not only younger generations but also senior citizens in adopting a healthier, more fulfilling lifestyle.

This book is the culmination of two months of his dedication, alongside his regular professional responsibilities. I feel honoured to have contributed to his manuscript and to share his wisdom with the world.

May Almighty God bless Dr. Shingari with excellent health and a long life to continue guiding his family, friends, and society.

—**Girish Kumar Vithal**

Editor

Foreword

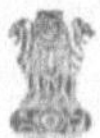 **Medical College, Baroda**
Vadodara, Gujarat, India.

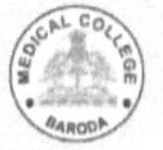

Dr. Vishwanath H. Chavali
Professor of Orthopaedics
Medical College, Baroda

FOREWORD

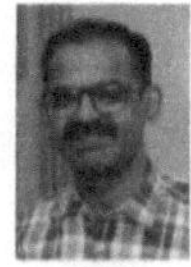

Aging is a universal journey, one that each of us will inevitably embark upon. Yet, the way we approach this journey can transform it into an experience of growth, resilience, and profound self-discovery. In *Genetic Threads: Navigating Confidence in the Fabric of Life*, Dr. M.K. Shingari offers a masterful exploration of the intricacies of aging, weaving together science, psychology, and spirituality into a guidebook for living gracefully beyond the age of 70. Dr. Shingari offers a roadmap for seniors to live fulfilling lives, regardless of their circumstances. It's an invaluable resource for both seniors and those who support them.

Dr. Shingari, drawing from his decades of personal and professional experience, presents aging not as a decline but as an opportunity to reflect, grow, and thrive. By emphasizing the interplay of genetics and environment, he highlights the aspects of our lives we can shape, empowering readers to take control of their health, mindset, and relationships. This book is not merely a study of aging but a call to action—a reminder that with preparation, positivity, and purpose, we can redefine what it means to grow older.

What sets this work apart is its practical relevance. Each chapter brims with actionable advice, from pre-retirement planning to fostering social connections, embracing spirituality, and understanding the transformative power of positive psychology. By addressing the emotional and existential aspects of aging, the book creates a holistic framework for readers to navigate this phase of life with dignity and grace. Real-life case studies, drawn from both India and abroad, illustrate the profound truths of this book in relatable, human terms.

As a society, we often view aging through the lens of limitations. Dr. Shingari challenges this perception, instead offering a vision of aging that is rich with possibilities. He inspires us to embrace this chapter of life as a time for renewal, learning, and giving back to the world in meaningful ways.

For anyone navigating their later years—or supporting a loved one through theirs—*Genetic Threads* is a beacon of hope and wisdom. It is an essential companion for anyone seeking to transform the inevitable process of aging into an enriching and fulfilling journey.

Warm regards,

Dr. Viswanath H. Chavali

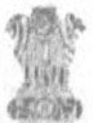

Medical College, Baroda
Vadodara, Gujarat, India.

BOOK REVIEW

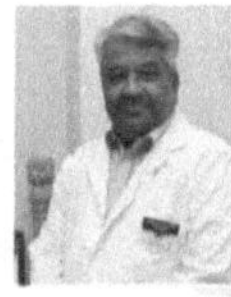

Aging is a natural part of life that brings both challenges and opportunities. In *Genetic Threads: Navigating Confidence in the Fabric of Life*, Dr. M.K. Shingari presents a thoughtful and comprehensive exploration of how individuals can approach their later years with purpose, resilience, and fulfillment.

One of the book's core messages is the importance of preparation. Dr. Shingari emphasizes that planning for retirement is about more than financial security—it's about developing hobbies, maintaining relationships, and creating a routine that fosters mental and physical well-being. By addressing these aspects early, individuals can build a foundation for a fulfilling post-retirement life.

The book also explores the interplay between genetics and environment in shaping our aging process. While we may inherit certain traits from our genes, the environment we cultivate—through our choices, relationships, and mindset—plays an equally significant role. This empowering perspective encourages readers to focus on factors they can control to improve their quality of life.

Dr. Shingari's emphasis on positive psychology offers a refreshing perspective on aging. Practices such as cultivating gratitude, building resilience, and staying socially connected are highlighted as essential tools for maintaining mental health and happiness. Real-life examples illustrate these principles in action, showcasing how individuals have overcome loneliness, health challenges, and other obstacles to rediscover confidence and joy in their later years.

The book also addresses societal and structural aspects of aging, such as the role of community support systems, government programs, and evolving family dynamics. By discussing these broader factors, the book offers readers a holistic view of how aging can be supported at both personal and societal levels.

Spirituality is another key theme, with the book emphasizing its importance in providing meaning and comfort during life's later stages. Whether through mindfulness, meditation, or a sense of connection to something larger than oneself, Dr. Shingari encourages readers to explore practices that can bring peace and resilience as they navigate aging's complexities.

Overall, *Genetic Threads* is more than a guide to aging—it's a call to embrace this phase of life with curiosity and confidence. Dr. Shingari's insights, combined with practical advice and relatable stories, make this book a valuable resource for seniors and their families. It redefines aging as a time of growth, self-discovery, and meaningful connection, offering hope and guidance for anyone looking to live fully at every stage of life.

Dr. Ranjan Aiyer
Professor of Otorhinolaryngology
Medical Superintendent, SSG Hospital

Vadodara, Gujarat

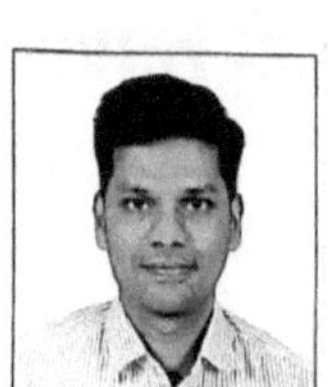

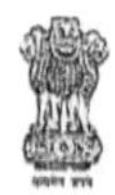

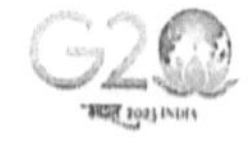

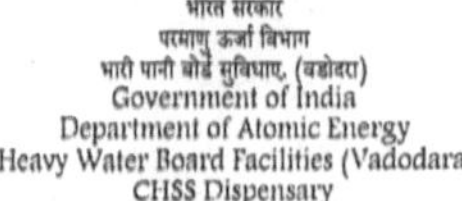

भारत सरकार
परमाणु ऊर्जा विभाग
भारी पानी बोर्ड सुविधाएं, (वड़ोदरा)
Government of India
Department of Atomic Energy
Heavy Water Board Facilities (Vadodara)
CHSS Dispensary

डाकघर, फर्टिलाइजरनगर
जिला, वड़ोदरा- 391750
P.O., Fertilizernagar
Dist., Vadodara- 391750

Dr. G. Pavan Kumar
Medical Officer Incharge
Heavy Water Board Facility, Vadodara

Book Review

In this modern era with ever evolving technology, increasing population, pollut bridization and processing of food and food products and people leading sedentary and sophistic estyle in isolated nuclear families with stress- people are landing up in disease like Diab ypertension /Obesity / Cardiovascular diseases etc.

A constant, Continuous and Sincere effort is required by every individua ercome such preventable diseases. Younger generation should adapt to Healthy Lifestyle, avoid j od and processed food, maintain ideal BODY MASS INDEX (BMI) and adapt to one Spor lividual choice according to their personality to stay Fit, Happy and Healthy.

Dr. Shingari Sir, an eminent personality of 85 years, had set himself as a live exan how to balance an individual's life academically and professionally and a balance between blen lotions like family relation, friends, stress management and devotion through disciplined lifestyle

The way Dr. Shingari Sir had compiled the difficulties faced by Senior citizens in er half of their life and the preparation to be made to overcome all such difficulties and lea ppy, Healthy and Successful Post Retirement Life through this book "Genetic Threads" This b worth reading not only to the Senior citizens but to All the Younger generation which gives eno ifidence, and ray of hope for people who wish to plan for a better future.

lso would request everyone to follow **"Lifestyle."**

Limit salt & Alcohol
nclude daily calcium and Potassium
ight fat and cholesterol
Exercise regularly
Stress Management
Try to Quit Smoking
Your medicine to be taken regularly
Loose weight maintain ideal BMI
End stage complication to be avoided

(Dr. G. Pavan Kumar)

An Open Letter to Super Seniors

A Call for Proper Pre-planning and a Revised Approach to Retirement Life

Dear Esteemed Seniors,

As I approach the 85th year of my life, with over 25 years of experience in observing the lives of senior and super-senior citizens across our country, I feel compelled to share my thoughts on the importance of **pre-planning for retirement** and how it can profoundly impact your quality of life in these later years.

Many people nearing retirement—often just 1 or 2 years before they officially retire—are occupied with worries about what life will look like without their office chair, their colleagues, or the status they once held in their professional lives. The fear of a future to be spent in idleness, with nothing to do but watch television or scroll through social media, can be overwhelming.

I have seen first-hand how this uncertainty can quickly lead to depression. After 1 or 2 years of retirement, many individuals begin to feel lost. They don't know how to structure their time, how to stay mentally and physically engaged, or how to continue feeling useful. Some even feel the tension of interfering with domestic affairs at home, as family members and household help manage the household differently than the work/office environment. This can cause stress, frustration, and a sense of isolation. Instead of relishing retirement, they inadvertently end up facing a life full of difficulties.

In this letter, I aim to emphasize the importance of proper **pre-retirement planning**, as well as a structured approach to your daily life once retirement arrives. The shift from an active work life to retirement can be mentally upsetting, especially when one finds themselves with large stretches of free time. Without a plan, it's all too easy to become disengaged from life, leading to frustration and an unhealthy dependence on family or the home environment.

I strongly recommend to develop hobbies or interests during your working years that can be continued, or perhaps even expanded upon, after retirement. Whether it's reading, gardening, painting, playing music, volunteering, visiting temples or participating in social functions, **staying mentally active and physically engaged is very crucial.** These activities will not only give you a sense of purpose but will also help to keep you connected with the outside world, maintaining your mental health and overall well-being.

Retirement doesn't have to mean isolation. It can be an exciting time to explore new passions, build deeper relationships with friends and family, and even give back to society through volunteer work or community involvement. Participating in social gatherings or local events can keep you connected and make you feel a part of something larger than yourself, keeping loneliness and depression away from you.

Additionally, being actively involved in the household can offer a sense of contribution, but it requires balance. It's important to recognize that the dynamics of home life are different from those of the workplace. Family members and domestic helpers have their own roles and expectations, which may not always align with the way things worked at the office. <u>Understanding these differences and respecting the boundaries in family life will not only ease your own transition into retirement but will also contribute to a friendly and peaceful home environment.</u>

In conclusion, I urge all senior citizens to take these seriously and implement in their life. Retirement should be a time of fulfillment, not of stagnation. With thoughtful pre-planning and an openness to exploring new activities, you can ensure that your retired life is not only productive but also deeply satisfying. The key is to keep learning, keep socializing, and keep moving forward.

Retirement is a gift—make the most of it.

Warm regards,

—Dr. M.K. Shingari

Introduction

Aging is an inevitable and gradual process that brings with it profound changes across various aspects of life. These changes, while natural, can be challenging and may impact one's Physical, Emotional, and Mental well-being. Common signs of aging include wrinkles, gray hair, and changes to the heart, teeth, eyes, and ears. The most notable change in the cardiovascular system is the stiffening of blood vessels and arteries, which causes the heart to work harder to pump blood. As we age, bones, joints, and muscles tend to shrink in size and density, which, along with weakening, can sometimes also lead to a decrease in height. Age-related changes can affect the digestive system as well, particularly in the large intestine. Furthermore, the bladder and urinary tract may lose elasticity, resulting in more frequent urination.

Cognitive functions, such as memory and thinking skills, also undergo changes, which may manifest as forgetfulness, such as forgetting familiar names or simple tasks. In addition, changes in vision and hearing are common. Eyes become less effective at focusing, glare sensitivity increases, and cataracts may develop, impairing vision. Hearing also tends to decline, making it harder to hear certain sounds or conversations.

Though these changes are often considered inevitable, they don't define the experience of aging. With a better understanding of the biological, psychological, and social factors at play, we can navigate the challenges of aging with resilience and confidence. My own journey, as well as the experiences of many friends and fellow seniors, has shown me that 'Aging need not mean a decline in overall quality of life'. Through proper care, a positive mindset, and the right lifestyle choices, it is possible to maintain health, vitality, and independence well into older age.

I, Dr. Mahendra Kumar Shingari, 85 years of age, hold a Ph.D. in Chemical Engineering from the United Kingdom. I have lived through the various transitions that come with aging, experiencing both the difficulties and the joys of each life stage. Many of my friends and fellow senior citizens, even those approaching the age of 60, face challenges such as memory loss, joint pain, and limited independence. I am fortunate to have had the guidance of many doctor friends from various specialties, who have provided valuable tips throughout my life on how to stay healthy and stress-free. Additionally, I have always been diligent about following these recommendations and studying scientific literature to understand their importance. I am also grateful to my grandparents and parents, who instilled discipline and a positive attitude, which have become central to my lifestyle.

This book is born from the encouragement of friends who suggested I share my experiences and the lifestyle practices that I believe contribute to aging with good health. Their support led me to delve into various scientific texts and organize my thoughts on how to maintain vitality even after 70. The purpose of this book is to explore the multifaceted effects of aging, particularly the physical and mental challenges such as memory loss, chronic pain, and sleep disturbances. We will also examine the emotional impact these changes can have, especially as we reach the age of 70 and beyond.

However, aging does not have to mean a decline in well-being. With the right mindset, it can be a period of growth, reflection, and renewal. Central to this process is the concept of positive psychology—a field that emphasizes nurturing optimism, resilience, and life satisfaction. These qualities are crucial for overcoming the challenges of aging and living a fulfilling life in later years. **How one perceives aging—whether with acceptance or resistance—plays a significant role in shaping the experience of these years.**

In the following chapters, I will explore the interplay between Genetics (our inherent traits) and the Environment (the experiences and nurturing that shape us) in determining how we age. I will also discuss the importance of emotional well-being, social connections, and spiritual growth as we advance in years. Through case studies from different parts of the world, **I will illustrate how individuals experience aging in diverse ways, and how self-confidence—both personal and collective—affects overall well-being.**

This book will feature six documented case studies: three from European countries and the USA, and three from India. These cases highlight the varied ways in which people experience aging, showcasing how their self-confidence plays a critical role in their quality of life. Additionally, real-life examples from our family and friends will demonstrate the different ways aging is navigated. **These experiences were instrumental in motivating me to compile my observations, knowledge, and lifelong lessons into this book.**

In conclusion, while the insights and suggestions provided throughout this book will be beneficial to the readers, the guidance in Chapter 11 and Appendices will be particularly valuable to those in their 70s and beyond.

This book will also be very useful for people in 50's to properly plan how they should mentally prepare themselves for better lifestyle after their retirement to keep them happy and satisfied.

I am sure that this book will offer both Practical advice and Emotional support, helping individuals—especially younger ones—to adopt healthier lifestyles and embrace the later years of life with confidence, wisdom, and joy.

***

Chapter 2

Aging and it's Side Effects

In this chapter, we examine the physical changes that occur with ageing, from minor discomforts like dry skin and aching joints to more serious health issues such as heart disease, diabetes, and memory loss. Ageing can bring both challenges and wisdom. We will discuss common age-related issues, including reduced mobility, sensory impairments (such as hearing and vision), and chronic conditions. The chapter will also address the emotional and psychological impact of these physical changes, which can often lead to feelings of frustration or getting lost.

As people grow older, they often say things like, "My energy is not what it used to be," or "Old age is catching up with me." I have heard this from friends and others in my community. When I hear these comments, I remind them **"Age is just a number"**. For example, I am 85 years old, but I do not feel that my intelligence, or focus is getting worse but my energy level has reduced. Many of my friends agree that I look just as energetic as I did 40 or 50 years ago, but I know that my energy level and stamina has decreased. Yes, our bodies change as we age, but there are many things like our **genes**, **environment**, and **education**, that can help keep us healthy and sharp.

Aging changes occur in all of the body's cells, tissues, and organs, and these changes affect the functioning of all body systems. Living tissue is made up of cells. Tissues are layers of similar cells that perform a specific function. The different kinds of tissues group together to form organs.

As aging continues, waste products build up in tissue which starts becoming more stiff. This makes the organs, blood vessels, and airways more rigid. Cell membranes change, so many tissues have more trouble getting oxygen and nutrients and removing carbon dioxide and other wastes. Many tissues lose mass. Some tissues become lumpy (nodular) or more rigid.

Because of cell and tissue changes, your organs also change as you age. Aging organs slowly lose function. Most of you do not notice this loss immediately, because you rarely need to use your organs to their fullest ability.

Organs have a reserve ability to function beyond the usual needs. **For example, the heart of a 20-year-old is capable of pumping about 10 times the amount of blood that is actually needed to keep the body alive. After age 30, an average of 1% of this reserve is lost each year.** The biggest changes in organ reserve occur in the heart, lungs, and kidneys. The amount of reserve lost varies between people and between different organs in a single person.

These changes appear slowly and over a long period. When an organ is worked harder than usual, it may not be able to increase function. Sudden heart failure or other problems can develop when the body is worked harder than usual. Loss of reserve also makes it harder to restore balance (equilibrium) in the body. Drugs are removed from the body by the kidneys and liver at a slower rate. Lower doses of medicines may be needed, to reduce the side effects. Recovery from illnesses is seldom 100%, leading to more and more disability. Side effects of medicine can mimic the symptoms of many diseases, so it is easy to mistake a drug reaction for an illness.

Why difference in Aging of different individuals

No one knows how and why people change as they get older. Some theories claim that aging is caused by injuries from ultraviolet light over time, wear and tear on the body, or by-product's of metabolism. Other theories view aging as a predetermined process controlled by genes. No single process can explain all the changes of aging. Aging is a complex process that varies as to how it affects different people and even different organs. Although some changes always occur with aging, they occur at different rates and to different extents. There is no way to predict exactly how you will age.

Most Gerontologists (people who study aging) feel that aging is due to the interaction of many lifelong influences. These influences include heredity, environment, culture,

diet, exercise & leisure, past illnesses, and many other factors. Unlike the changes of adolescence, which are predictable to within a few years, each person ages at a unique rate. Some systems begin aging as early as age 30. Other aging processes are not common until much later in life.

This brings us to an important question: **How do our genes (nature) and our environment (nurturing) affect the way we live and age?** This has been a topic of discussion for many years. Some people believe we are mostly shaped by our genes, while others think our environment—like our upbringing, education, and life experiences—has a bigger impact. In reality, it's a mix of both. **Our genes can influence how we look** or how our bodies work, but our education, experiences, choices, and the people around us also play a big role. This mix of **Nature and Nurture** continues to shape us throughout our lives.

I am sharing some case studies to show how different people, in both developed and developing countries, are affected by their experiences as they age.

Case Studies on Aging and Confidence

CASE 1: Memory Loss and Confidence (UK)

Alice Spencer, an 82-year-old woman from England, was known for her sharp mind and sense of humour. She had been a school teacher for over 40 years and continued to tutor children even after retirement. But over the time, **she started forgetting** things—small things at first, like where she put her keys. Later, she began forgetting bigger things, like which plants to prune in her garden.

One day, Alice realized she couldn't remember how to make her favourite chicken pot pie, a recipe she'd cooked many times. She felt upset and worried. Her daughter, Susan, noticed these changes and suggested they see a Doctor who **diagnosed Alice with early-stage Alzheimer's disease.** Alice was afraid of becoming a burden to her family, and her confidence began to fade. She stopped tutoring, withdrew from social activities, and even struggled with daily tasks.

But **Susan didn't give up**. She helped Alice cook, reminding her of old memories and encouraging her to keep going. Over the time, Alice joined a support group for people with memory problems. With her family's support, Alice returned to teaching children, this time with help. Slowly, she regained some of her confidence and found joy in being with others, even if she needed reminders and help.

Lesson: Memory loss is a tough challenge, but with love, support, and understanding, confidence can be rebuilt even in the face of Alzheimer's disease.

CASE 2: Shrinking Social Circle and Confidence (USA)

Walter Thompson, an 85-year-old retired Engineer, used to have a wide circle of friends and loved socializing. But as he got older, many of his friends no longer around or passed away. His own health problems made it harder for him to leave the house, and he spent more time alone, relying mostly on his daughter, Karen, for companionship. Walter's confidence began to fade as his world grew smaller.

One day, Karen suggested him to join a local senior group. Walter felt unsure and worried as he wouldn't fit in. He was afraid he wouldn't be as sharp as others and would be judged for his age. But when Karen brought over an old friend, Henry, to visit, Walter realized he still had valuable friendships. This visit sparked his confidence.

Eventually, Walter joined the senior group and started attending weekly meetings. At first, it was awkward, but over the time, he made new friends and began to enjoy the conversations. He even volunteered to lead a discussion group. Slowly, Walter's confidence returned. He realized that it's never too late to make new connections and that socializing can bring joy and confidence, even in old age.

Lesson: Having a strong social circle and being open to new connections helps maintain confidence, especially when old friends are no longer around.

CASE 3: Inherited Strength and Confidence (UK)

Lena Mitchell, a 28-year-old medical student, often felt unsure about herself, despite her many achievements.

She came from a family with a history of mental health struggles—her grandmother had battled severe depression and her father dealt with anxiety and low self-esteem. Lena feared she might inherit these struggles.

Lena confided in her mentor, Dr. Harris, who encouraged her to focus on her strengths rather than her family's history. With his help, Lena learned to manage her anxiety and build her confidence. Over the time, she began to see her family history as something that had shaped her into a more compassionate and resilient person, not something that defined her. By the end of medical school, Lena had gained enough confidence to become a skilled and compassionate Doctor.

Lesson: Our family history might affect us, but we can choose how we respond to it. Understanding our heritage can give us strength but should not limit us.

CASE 4: The Power of Social Circles in Old Age (India)

Rajiv Kumar, a retired school Principal from Mumbai, felt lonely after his wife passed away. His children lived abroad, and many of his old friends had moved away. Rajiv began to feel isolated and his confidence reduced.

One of his neighbour, Mrs. Gupta, noticed his loneliness and invited him to tea. She then organized regular meetings for the elderly people in the neighbourhood. At first, Rajiv was reluctant, but as he attended these meetings, he began to feel more connected. He even started volunteering at a local orphanage and leading activities for the children.

Through these new social interactions, Rajiv regained his confidence. He realized that being around people who cared about him and shared similar experiences, could bring joy and purpose, even in old age.

Lesson: In many societies, especially in India, having a supportive social circle can significantly improve the confidence and well-being of elderly people. Regular social connections can reduce loneliness and provide a sense of living.

CASE 5: The Influence of Education, Culture, and Family on Confidence (Pakistan)

This is the story of Aamir, a man from Karachi, Pakistan, who is now in his 70's. He often reflects on his life journey, especially as he watches his grandchildren grow and face their own challenges.

Aamir grew up in a modest neighbourhood. His family wasn't wealthy, but they believed strongly in the power of education. His father was a teacher, and his mother was a homemaker who took great pride in their culture. Every evening, after helping his mother with chores, Aamir would sit with his father and together they would read books and discuss different subjects. His father's love for learning was contagious, and Aamir developed a deep interest in gaining knowledge.

But it wasn't just his education that shaped him. Aamir's family also held on to their cultural traditions. They valued Urdu poetry, Sufi music, and the principles of hospitality. Aamir's grandmother often told him stories about heroes and wise people from their culture, which made him proud of his heritage.

Despite not having much money, Aamir's family always found ways to support his education. Aamir worked hard and earned a scholarship to attend a University, where he studied with students from wealthier families who spoke English fluently. At first, Aamir felt out of place and unsure of himself. But he remembered the advice his father had given him: *"Knowledge is your strength, and your culture is your anchor."* He also thought of his mother, who was strong and proud of their traditions. These thoughts helped Aamir stay confident, and he worked hard to succeed.

After finishing his studies, Aamir became a respected professor at the same University. He taught not only academic subjects but also shared wisdom about his culture. He made sure to mentor students from poorer backgrounds, just like he had once been, encouraging them to be proud of their roots and to see their heritage as a source of strength.

Now, in his old age, Aamir's confidence is still strong. He is admired by his community and often invited to speak at cultural events and educational seminars. His children and grandchildren look up to him, not only as the head of the family but as an example of how education, culture, and family support can shape someone's life and confidence.

One evening, while sitting with his grandchildren, Aamir recited a famous couplet by Allama Iqbal, one of Pakistan's greatest poet:

"Khudi ko kar buland itna, खुदी को कर बुलंद इतना

Ke har taqdeer se pehle, के हर तक़दीर से पेहले,

Khuda bande se khud poochhe खुदा बंदे से खुद पुछे,

"Bata, teri raza kya hai?" "बता, तेरी रज़ा क्या है?"

 Meaning

"Elevate yourself to such heights that before every destiny, God Himself asks you, what is it that you desire?"

Lesson: Aamir felt proud as he spoke those words. He realized that the values his family had instilled in him had not only shaped his own life but would also continue to inspire his children and grandchildren for generations.

CASE 6: Swami Vivekananda's Quote on the Power of Thoughts

This story is about two brothers who were nurtured in the same home, but ended up leading very different lives. One became a successful businessman and the other struggled with addiction and unhealthy habits. People wanted to understand why these two brothers, who had the same parents and grew up in the same environment, turned out so differently.

The first brother, who became an alcoholic and a drug addict, was asked, *"Why do you live like this? Why do you harm yourself and your family?"* He answered, *"My father was a drug addict, a drunk, and he used to beat our family. That's what I saw growing up, so that's what I became."*

They then asked the second brother, who was successful and respected in the community, *"How did you turn out so well? What motivated you to make good choices?"* He replied, *"My father. I saw how he ruined his life with drinking and drugs. I promised myself that I would never be like him. I worked hard to be different, and now I'm proud of who I've become."*

This story shows that both brothers faced the same challenges growing up. They both had the same father, but one brother chose to follow in his father's footsteps, while the other chose to rise above it. Both brothers used their father's example as motivation, but one used it in a negative way, while the other used it to inspire positive change in his life.

Moral of the Story

The two brothers show how powerful our thoughts and mind-set can be. One chose to think that he was bound by his father's bad habits, and so he followed them. The other brother chose to think that he could make better choices, and his life was shaped by that positive thinking.

In life, our thoughts are incredibly important. If we focus on positive thoughts and strive to improve, we can change the course of our lives, no matter what was our past or the challenges we face.

Conclusion

These stories teach us important lessons about ageing, memory, mental health, and the factors that shape who we are.

Alice's story shows how a **supportive family** and resilience can help us deal with memory loss.

Walter's story teaches us that **social connections** are crucial in maintaining confidence and happiness as we age.

Lena's experience demonstrates that while our **genes influence** us, they don't control our fate. We can change our destiny with the right mind-set.

Rajiv's story emphasizes the **power of community** and the support of friends in later years.

Swami Vivekanand quote teaches us that our thoughts are incredible important for guiding our life.

Aamir story highlights how the values installed by the parents shape up individual's life.

Chapter 3

Nature (Genes) vs Nurture

(Environmental Influences)

Understanding Nature vs. Nurture: A Path for Better Living for Seniors Around 70

This chapter delves into the longstanding debate of whether our Genetics (Nature) or our upbringing and life Experiences (Nurture) have a greater impact on who we are, especially as we age. If twins are raised in different environments, we may see that even with identical genetic makeup they may develop different personalities. Let's explore both aspects, Nature and Nurture, and their roles in shaping our personalities, health, and behaviour as we grow older.

What Do Nature and Nurture Mean?

Nature refers to the Genetic traits we inherit from our parents, influencing our personality, intelligence, physical characteristics, and some aspects of behaviour.

Nurture, on the other hand, is the influence of our environment—family, education, social conditions, culture, and experiences—that shapes our behaviour and personal development.

Historically, it was believed that we were born as "blank slates," with our environment alone shaping us. However, as research in genetics advanced, it became clear that we come into the world with certain genetic instructions that influence our growth and behaviour. Our genes set the foundation, but it is the environment that helps us develop into who we are.

The Balance Between Nature and Nurture

After decades of research, most experts agree that both genetics and environment play equal roles in shaping who we become—about 50% each. This means that while your genes give you certain traits and predispositions, your experiences and the environment around you significantly influence your health, behaviour, and overall aging process.

Practical Experience and Observations

From personal experience, especially over the last 60 years of observing family, friends, neighbour, and senior citizens, it is clear that the **environment** plays a huge role in shaping a person's personality.

For example, after the **Partition of India in 1947**, many families, including mine, had to leave what is now Pakistan and move to India. These families lost everything — their homes, belongings, and wealth — and arrived in Delhi or other cities with nothing. They were living in refugee camps or temporary shelters, having to start life from scratch.

Among the refugees, there were two types of people:

Older people, who had lived a comfortable life before the Partition and were then struggling to find work to survive. They had to adapt quickly to very difficult conditions.

Younger people, many of whom were well-educated professionals or students, determined to rebuild their lives. However, they faced a harsh new reality and had to make quick decisions for survival. Some resorted to dishonest and illegal activities, such as selling adulterated food or engaging in violence, just to make money.

This shift in behaviour was not just about their personal choices but due to **environmental stress** they were facing. The refugee crisis affected their thinking and actions. This environment of hardship and survival led to a cycle where unscrupulous practices became more common in the migrated community. **This shift in behaviour and values, driven by the environmental conditions and the desperate circumstances of the post-Partition period,**

created a culture where unscrupulous practices became the norm.

As the years passed, the next generation continued these behaviours, and it became part of the culture of the city.

This phenomenon was widespread among the refugee population. Many of them, who had once been the cream of society, **became prosperous again through these dubious means.** However, their practices had far-reaching consequences, influencing not just their immediate environment but also the broader culture of the city. **The next generation inherited these survival tactics, perpetuating a cycle of corruption and moral compromise.**

As a result, the cultural landscape of, as an example, Delhi underwent a significant transformation. The city became known for its high levels of violence, pervasive cheating, and a general atmosphere of distrust. People became short-tempered and quick to resort to aggression.

Therefore, for those who wish to live honest and simple lives in Delhi is often perceived as an unsafe place. The legacy of that tumultuous period continues to influence the city's culture, making it a place where making money often trumps ethical considerations.

Genetics and Intelligence

When it comes to intelligence, it is important to understand that it is not controlled by just one **"intelligence gene"**.

Instead, intelligence is the result of many **genes working together** (called "polygenic").

For example, if a person has tall parents, it's likely that they may also be tall. But factors like nutrition, health, and overall care during childhood can affect just how tall they become. If a child has one tall parent and one short parent, the child's height normally may fall somewhere between the two parents' heights.

In the same way, **intelligence** can be influenced by a combination of genetic factors and environmental factors. Research has shown that intelligence is not just about what you are born with but also about how you grow up, the education you get, and the environment you are in.

For instance:

Identical twins raised in different homes tend to have slightly different IQs, even though they share the same genetics.

Children who are **breastfed** for longer periods tend to have higher IQs when they reach adulthood.

Vitamin and nutrient deficiencies during childhood can also lower IQ levels later in life.

First-Born Children and Intelligence

Studies show that **first-born children** often have **higher IQs** than their younger siblings. This may be because they get more attention from their parents, and there are higher expectations for them to succeed.

However, in my experience (having observed families for over 60 years), the reality can be more complex. **First-born children** often feel the pressure of being the "experiment" for their parents. They might receive a lot of love, but also a lot of expectations and discipline. This can leave them feeling stressed and uncertain about themselves.

On the other hand, **younger siblings** might benefit from their parents' **more relaxed approach**, as their parents have learned from their earlier experiences with the first child. This can create a different family dynamic, where the first-born feels like a role model, while the younger siblings might have a more balanced upbringing.

This example highlights how powerful the environment can be in shaping not only individuals but entire communities, and how circumstances of survival can affect moral choices and long-term behaviour.

Mental Health: The Role of Nature and Nurture

When it comes to mental health, both genetic factors and life experiences contribute. Some mental health conditions, like depression or schizophrenia, can run in families, showing a genetic influence. However, environmental stressors like work pressure, trauma, loss, or substance abuse can trigger these conditions. Therapy can address both environmental factors (such as past trauma) and the genetic components (such as brain chemistry) to improve mental health.

What can Seniors do to Improve their Lives?

For seniors around 70, understanding the balance between nature and nurture can be empowering. It shows that while we may not be able to change our genetic makeup, we have significant control over how our environment shapes us. Here are some practical steps for better living:

Adapt to Change: Embrace the changes that come with aging. Seek help when needed, and stay flexible in adjusting to new health or social challenges.

Focus on Positive Environments: Surround yourself with supportive people, engage in activities that stimulate your mind, and create a peaceful and enriching living space.

Engage in Lifelong Learning: Never stop exploring new ideas, hobbies, or skills. Studies show that continuous learning can help maintain cognitive function and improve mental well-being.

Prioritize Physical and Mental Health: Eat nutritious food, exercise regularly, and engage in social activities. Positive lifestyle choices can significantly impact how you age.

Intergenerational Conversations: Talk to younger generations about how the world has changed over time. Share wisdom and encourage them to think about how their environment will shape their lives, just as yours has shaped yours.

Explore Mental Health: Reflect on how mental health challenges are handled in your community. Consider how your upbringing or personal experiences have shaped your approach to mental health, and explore different therapy options if needed.

Conclusion

Ultimately, both Nature and Nurture work together throughout our lives. While we can't change our genetic makeup, we can influence our environment to create a healthier, happier, and more fulfilling life as we age.

Chapter 4

Positive Psychology and Aging

(Understanding the Influence of Positive Psychology on Behaviour and Well-Being in Seniors)

Introduction

*"It is not the years in your life that count,
it is the life in your years."*

—Adlai Stevenson

Aging is a natural part of the human experience, but as individuals grow older, particularly around 70, they often face physical, emotional, and psychological challenges. The field of positive psychology, which focuses on promoting well-being, strengths, and flourishing, offers valuable insights into how seniors can navigate the aging process with resilience and vitality. In this chapter, I explore the role of positive psychology in aging, how psychology influences behaviour in individuals over the age of 70, the impact of negative psychology on older adults, and how negative psychological states can be avoided. I will also suggest lifestyle changes that can promote a healthy, fulfilling, and active life for seniors.

The Role of Positive Psychology in Aging

Positive psychology refers to the study of how we can best function and promote human flourishing. Positive psychology is a science that brings many virtues of science and science has proven that stress is directly linked with our immune system. This means **our bodies are more susceptible to bacterial and viral attacks if we have endure stress and/or other negative experiences.**

Positive psychology, focuses on strengths, virtues, and factors that contribute to an individual's happiness, life satisfaction, and personal development. It encourages people to focus not only on their challenges but also on what they can do to enhance their lives. For older adults, embracing positive psychology can significantly improve their mental health, sense of purpose, and overall quality of life. The aims of positive psychology are:.

- Rise to life's challenges, and make the most out of setbacks

- Engage with other people to build positive relationships

- Find fulfillment in creativity and productivity

- Help others to find peace and satisfaction.

- In the context of aging, positive psychology emphasizes:

Gratitude and Acceptance: Seniors who practice gratitude tend to have better emotional well-being and more positive relationships. By focusing on the positives in their lives, such as their achievements and the love they've experienced, they can cultivate an optimistic outlook.

Resilience: Aging can bring about loss—whether it is the death of friends or within family, physical decline or the loss of independence. Positive psychology helps individuals develop resilience, enabling them to bounce back from adversity and overcome these challenges.

Engagement: Positive psychology suggests that individuals are happiest when fully engaged in activities they enjoy. For seniors, finding hobbies, volunteering, or learning new skills can lead to a sense of accomplishment and purpose.

Social Connections: Strong social support is a critical factor in aging well. Positive psychology emphasizes the importance of building and maintaining meaningful relationships, which have been linked to reduced rates of depression and cognitive decline in older adults.

Psychological Effects on Behaviour in Older Adults

The psychological state of older adults significantly influences their behaviour and overall life satisfaction. **As people enter their 70s and beyond, they often undergo shifts in their mental and emotional states due to a combination of physiological, social, and environmental factors.** Some of the key psychological effects include:

Changes in Cognitive Functioning: Aging often comes with a decline in cognitive abilities viz. Mental processes that take place in the brain, including thinking, attention, language, learning, memory and perception. However, research suggests that cognitive decline can be reduced by positive psychological factors like engagement in mentally stimulating activities. Lifelong learning, puzzles, and creative hobbies (such as painting or writing) help maintain cognitive function and contribute to a greater sense of self-worth.

Increased Emotional Regulation: Interestingly, many older adults report feeling more emotionally balanced and less reactive than in their younger years. This phenomenon is linked to increased emotional regulation that comes with age. Older adults are often better at letting go of minor irritations and focusing on what truly matters, which contributes to greater life satisfaction and fewer emotional disturbances.

Motivation and Purpose: **After the age of 70, individuals often retire from work, which can cause a loss of identity and purpose for some.** However, those who have developed a strong sense of meaning in life are better able to transition into this new phase. Positive psychology highlights the importance of developing a sense of purpose, whether through volunteering, mentoring, pursuing hobbies, or spending time with family. A strong sense of purpose (Clear reasons for what you want to do) has been linked to improved mental and physical health outcomes in older adults.

Social Behaviour and Isolation: Social engagement tends to decline as people age due to factors like mobility limitations, the experience of losing someone important, or changes in social roles. However, staying socially connected is vital for emotional well-being. Seniors who continue to engage in social activities, such as family gatherings, social clubs, or community events, tend to experience lower rates of depression, anxiety, and loneliness.

I would like to site a real example to highlight the effect of proper pre- retirement planning. My friend Mr. Girish Kumar Vithal who was General Manager in Heavy Water Board, Mumbai, a unit of Department of Atomic Energy. I was frequently visiting him. He was staying in Departmental accommodation throughout. Basically he is Delhite but has a flat in Mumbai which was always on rent. Actually he had one daughter Mahima studying in B.E. but suffering from Autoimmune disorder. His wife Suneeta Vithal was lecturer in Junior College and has chronic health issues. This family was not interested in settling at Delhi because of severe climatic conditions and poor law and order situation there. They also wanted to have reasonable big flat to stay after retirement. He asked my opinion on where to settle down after retirement.

Seeing the attitude and family circumstances of Mr. Vithal, I advised him to settle in small city like Baroda / Mysore having good law and order with moderate climate and good medical facilities. As I am from Vadodara and knew that Mr. Vithal has two of his old colleagues of similar age posted in Heavy Water Plant Baroda and they planned to settle there itself inspite of being from different states, I, based on my experience, advised Mr. Vithal to settle in Vadodara with his friends.

Nowadays children mostly go for jobs either abroad or to different cities, most of the parents have to stay alone. My experience says that a good company of similar chemistry among families in the neighbourhood is very difficult, therefore friends who have been colleagues also for 4 decades staying together will be a very healthy and happy situation.

Mr. Vithal agreed to my suggestion and took a flat in the same big Housing Society where his other 2 colleagues had bought. Seeing him shifting from Mumbai even when Mr. Vithal has already a flat in Mumbai, his two other batchmates bought the flats in the same housing Society. Mr. Vithal is staying there for the last 9 years and always thank me for the practical advice as All the friends are very happy, daily meeting for walks, together celebrate birthdays and anniversary's of every family members and always available to physically and morally support each other on any occasion. He always says that they never feel that they are retired. All these families get special attention by the society residents and give suggestions where are required in various activities of the Society.

I am sure that readers will able to appreciate whatever is suggested for them will be very useful if they timely follow these.

The Impact of Negative Psychology on Older Adults

While positive psychology provides a framework for improving the well-being of older adults, negative psychology/negative attitudes will worsen the challenges that come with aging. Older people also have significant consequences for the physical and mental health. Older people who feel they are a burden and think that their lives to be less valuable, putting them at risk of depression and social isolation. Recently published research shows that older people who hold negative views about their own aging, do not recover as well from disability and live on an average 8 to 10 years less than people with positive attitudes.

Negative psychological states, such as depression, anxiety, and loneliness, can significantly affect behaviour and overall health in seniors. **If your senior loved one is becoming progressively more negative as they age, it may be due to diminished health, increased isolation, boredom, or other factors.**

Some factors that contribute to negative psychology in aging include:

Depression and Anxiety: Older adults may struggle with depression due to health problems, loss of loved ones, or the perceived loss of social status or independence. Anxiety may also arise from fears about death, financial insecurity, or health concerns. Left untreated, these negative psychological states can lead to social withdrawal, diminished motivation, and poorer physical health.

Cognitive Decline and Dementia: Cognitive decline, including conditions like Alzheimer's disease and other dementia, can also be aggravated by negative psychological states. Seniors who feel hopeless or fearful about their mental decline may be less likely to seek treatment or engage in cognitive exercises, leading to a further reduction in mental capacity.

Loneliness and Social Isolation: The loss of friends, family members, and not getting socially involved in day to day life, can lead to isolation and loneliness in older adults. Social isolation is a significant risk factor for mental health problems such as depression, and it can also accelerate physical health decline, contributing to conditions like heart disease and high blood pressure.

Avoiding Negative Psychology in Aging

To counter the negative effects of aging and avoid the pitfalls (unexpected events in life that sneak up on you and ruin your life's plan) of negative psychology, seniors can adopt a variety of strategies:

Building Resilience: Developing coping mechanisms for handling stress and loss is crucial for aging well. Seniors can focus on building their resilience through mindfulness, meditation, and cognitive-behavioral strategies. These techniques can help re-frame negative thoughts and promote a more positive outlook on life.

Maintaining Physical Health: Physical activity is not only important for physical well-being but also for mental health. Regular exercise has been shown to reduce symptoms of depression and anxiety, improve sleep, and boost cognitive function. It is important for seniors to stay active within their physical limits, whether it's through walking, **yoga or meditation but always under the guidance of trained teachers.**

Social Engagement: Staying connected to others is one of the most powerful tools in combating negative psychology. Seniors should make an effort to maintain relationships with family, friends, and their community. Technology, such as video calls, social media, and online communities, can also help seniors stay connected.

Seeking Professional Support: Mental health professionals, such as therapists or counselors, can be invaluable in helping seniors address feelings of sadness, anxiety, or loss. Therapy, particularly cognitive-behaviour therapy (CBT), can help seniors re-frame negative thoughts and build coping skills.

Suggested Lifestyle for Seniors Above 70's

The key to healthy aging lies in maintaining both physical and mental well-being. Positive psychology focuses on the **'Well–Being theory'**, which asserts that there are five components to lead a good life. These **five components** are key to how all of us can cultivate happier aging. These are **Positive Emotion, Engagement, Relationships, Accomplishments and Understanding meaning of life.**

Here are some lifestyle recommendations for seniors over 70's:

Regular Physical Activity: Engage in low-impact activities like walking, and deep breathing etc.. These activities improve cardiovascular health, flexibility, and strength while reducing the risk of chronic diseases like diabetes and arthritis.

Nutritious Diet: A balanced diet rich in vegetables, fruits, whole grains, and lean proteins supports both physical and cognitive health. Seniors should focus on nutrient-dense foods to maintain energy and reduce the risk of illness.

Mental Stimulation: Use of your mind with activities that require concentration and creativity, such as puzzles, reading, writing, or learning a new skill. These activities help maintain cognitive function and enhance self-esteem.

Building Meaningful Relationships: Cultivate social connections with family, friends, or local community groups. Engaging in social activities, whether online or in person, helps prevent loneliness and enriches life.

Emotional Health: Practice to pay attention, live in the present, treat yourself the way you would treat a good friend, focus on your breathing, meditation, or relaxation techniques to reduce stress and promote emotional well-being. Engaging in hobbies, volunteering, or pursuing personal passions can foster a sense of purpose.

Quality Sleep: Prioritize good sleep and schedule/ bedroom discipline to ensure that you feel healthier and stronger. A regular sleep schedule, a relaxing bedtime routine, and a comfortable sleep environment can improve overall well-being.

Conclusion

Aging is a multifaceted experience that involves both challenges and opportunities for growth. **Positive psychology offers a valuable framework for seniors to embrace the aging process with optimism, resilience, and fulfillment.** By focusing on their strengths, maintaining social connections, staying physically and mentally active, and developing coping/adjusting skills, seniors can enhance their quality of life and age with grace. Avoid negative psychological states. Ultimately, the way we approach aging, both mentally and physically, has a profound impact on how we live in our 70's and beyond.

Chapter 5

Mental Health and Well-Being in Old Age

A Focus on Individuals Aged around 70

As people age, their mental and emotional well-being become increasingly important aspects of overall health. Among individuals aged near 70, maintaining mental health can be a challenge, influenced by various physical, psychological, and social factors. The aging process is often associated with a range of changes—retirement, loss of loved ones, physical decline, and sometimes isolation—all of which can impact a person's mental health. However, with the right strategies and support, older adults can lead healthy, happy lives, preserving their mental and emotional well-being well into their later years.

Factors Affecting Mental Health in Older Adults

Several factors play a crucial role in shaping the mental health of older individuals. Physical health is one of the primary influences. Chronic conditions like arthritis, heart disease, or diabetes can lead to pain and discomfort, which in turn can cause stress, anxiety, or depression. Moreover, the process of aging often leads to a decline in mobility, and many older adults face challenges in completing everyday tasks. These factors can result in a diminished sense of autonomy and independence, leading to feelings of frustration, helplessness, or sadness.

Another factor affecting mental health in older adults is the loss of social connections. Retirement, relocation, or the death of friends and family members can lead to loneliness and isolation. Social interactions are key to maintaining mental health, and when these are reduced, the risk of developing mental health issues such as depression and anxiety increases. Additionally, the social stigma around aging can lead to a sense of invisibility or marginalization, contributing to negative self-perceptions and a decline in mental well-being.

Cognitive decline is also a significant concern for older adults. Conditions such as dementia or Alzheimer's disease affect memory, thinking, and behaviour, causing distress for both the individual and their loved ones. Cognitive decline can lead to confusion, frustration, and a loss of identity, which are all factors that can heavily impact mental health.

The Importance of Mental Health in Older Adults

Mental health is just as important as physical health, especially in older age. The well-being of individuals in their 70s and beyond can affect their quality of life, longevity, and even physical health outcomes. Depression and anxiety, for instance, have been linked to an increased risk of chronic diseases, such as heart disease, and can result in decreased immunity. Maintaining good mental health helps older adults remain independent, engage with their friends & relatives apart from the family members, and continue to enjoy the life.

Positive mental health also encourages resilience, helping older individuals to cope better with the inevitable challenges of aging, such as death of near and dear, chronic illness, or mobility limitations. It allows individuals to adapt to new circumstances, maintain a sense of purpose, and feel more connected to the world around them. In contrast, poor mental health can lead to a downward side, where negative emotions, such as sadness or anxiety, exacerbate physical symptoms and further reduce the quality of life.

Strategies to Promote Mental Health and Well-Being in Older Adults

To ensure that individuals in 70's maintain their mental health and well-being, a variety of strategies can be employed. These approaches focus on improving physical health, maintaining social connections, and promoting cognitive functioning.

Staying Physically Active: Regular physical activity is essential for mental health at any age, but it is particularly beneficial for older adults. Exercise releases endorphins, chemicals in the brain that boost mood, reduce stress, and increase feelings of happiness. Activities like walking, swimming, or yoga or meditation under the guidance of trained teachers can improve physical health, enhance mobility, and foster a sense of accomplishment. Moreover, regular exercise can reduce the risk of developing mental health conditions like depression and anxiety, and can even delay the onset of cognitive decline.

Engaging in Social Activities: Social connection is one of the most significant factors in maintaining mental health in older age. Engaging in social activities, whether it's joining a club, attending social events, or simply spending time with family and friends, can reduce feelings of isolation and provide emotional support. Social interactions stimulate the brain, foster a sense of belonging, and help individuals feel valued, all of which are crucial for maintaining a positive outlook on life.

Mindfulness and Stress Reduction: Mindfulness practices, such as meditation, deep breathing exercises, Super Brain Yoga exercises under the guidance of trained teachers, can significantly improve mental health by reducing stress and anxiety. These activities encourage individuals to focus on the present moment, helping them feel more grounded and less overwhelmed by the challenges of aging. Mindfulness has been shown to reduce symptoms of depression and improve cognitive function, making it an important tool for older adults.

Cognitive Exercises: Engaging in mentally stimulating activities such as reading, puzzles, learning new skills, or playing games can help keep the brain active and potentially delay the onset of cognitive decline. Lifelong learning and maintaining intellectual curiosity are associated with a decreased risk of developing conditions like dementia and Alzheimer's disease. Additionally, these activities provide a sense of purpose and fulfillment, which is key for emotional well-being.

Seeking Professional Support: If older individuals experience persistent feelings of sadness, anxiety, or hopelessness, seeking help from a mental health professional is crucial. Therapy, counselling, or support groups can provide valuable tools and coping strategies. There is no shame in seeking help as these behaviour changes are common in 70's. Mental health professionals are trained to address the unique challenges faced by older adults. Early intervention can prevent mental health issues from worsening and ensure a higher quality of life.

Conclusion

Mental health and well-being in older adults around 70 are integral to leading a happy, fulfilling life. Aging can bring about a range of challenges, from physical decline to loss of social connections, but with the right strategies in place, older individuals can maintain their mental health and continue to enjoy life. Staying physically active, engaging in social activities, practicing mindfulness, keeping the brain stimulated, and seeking professional help when needed are all essential steps to ensuring well-being in later years. By addressing these factors, older adults can face the challenges of aging with resilience, happiness, and a sense of purpose.

By opting above mentioned suggestions, senior adults can lead healthier, happier, and more fulfilling lives well into their later years.

Chapter 6

Spirituality and Aging

Spirituality often takes on a more prominent role as people age, providing a sense of meaning, purpose, and comfort. In this chapter, we will explore the importance of spirituality and how it can contribute to emotional and psychological resilience in old age. Whether through religion, meditation, or a personal sense of connection to the Universe, spirituality can offer elderly individuals a deeper sense of peace and help them navigate the transitions of aging.

Introduction

As people grow older, especially around 70, they face a range of physical, medical, and emotional challenges. These may include feelings of loneliness, fear of losing loved ones, or anxiety about death. Such challenges can affect their overall quality of life. Common issues include chronic health conditions, physical limitations, mental health problems, and social isolation. However, **spirituality** can provide a sense of purpose, inner peace, and strength, helping older adults navigate the difficulties of aging.

This chapter will explore the relationship between aging (which has already been defined in earlier chapters) and spirituality and how spiritual practices can support seniors in their later years.

Defining Spirituality

Spirituality is the sense of connection to something greater than oneself. It often involves seeking meaning, purpose, and inner peace. This connection may be expressed through religious practices, personal beliefs, or a broader understanding of life. Spirituality is not tied to any one religion but focuses on personal growth, mental balance, and emotional well-being.

Common Challenges Faced by Seniors around 70 Older adults face numerous challenges related to health, physical capabilities, mental well-being, and social and financial situations. These challenges can be grouped into the following categories:

1. Medical Problems

- **Chronic Diseases**: Seniors often have long-term health conditions such as arthritis, heart disease, diabetes, and respiratory issues that require ongoing care and affect daily activities.

- **Mobility Issues**: Conditions like osteoporosis, joint pain, and muscle weakness can limit mobility and increase the risk of falls, which can result in injury or disability.

- **Sensory Impairments**: Many older adults experience hearing loss or vision problems, leading to frustration, dependence, and social isolation.

2. Physical Challenges

- **Decreased Strength and Endurance**: Aging can lead to muscle weakness and lower stamina, making everyday tasks such as lifting objects or carrying groceries difficult.

- **Balance and Coordination Problems**: Weakened muscles and changes in the inner ear can impair balance and coordination, increasing the risk of falls and injuries.

- **Sleep Disorders**: Changes in sleep patterns, such as trouble falling or staying asleep, can cause fatigue, irritability, and poor health.

- **Nutritional Deficiencies**: Aging can affect appetite and digestion, making it harder to maintain a healthy diet, which may lead to weight loss and weakened immunity.

3. Mental Health Issues

- **Depression and Anxiety**: Many seniors experience mental health challenges, such as depression or anxiety, often triggered by physical decline, the loss of loved ones, or feelings of purposelessness.

- **Cognitive Decline**: Issues like forgetfulness, confusion, and difficulty with daily tasks are common, especially with Alzheimer's disease and dementia.

4. Social and Financial Challenges

- **Social Isolation**: As seniors age, they often lose close family and friends. Mobility issues may make it difficult to leave home and engage in social activities, contributing to isolation.

- **Financial Concerns**: Many seniors live on fixed incomes, such as pensions or Social Security, which may not be enough to cover healthcare costs and other expenses.

- **Intentionally postponing Healthcare**: Barriers such as financial limitations, mobility issues, or navigating complex insurance systems can delay necessary care.

5. End-of-Life Issues

- **Fear of Death**: Seniors often begin to confront their mortality, which can lead to fear, anxiety, or depression.

- **End-of-Life Decisions**: As health declines, seniors may need to make difficult decisions about their care, such as whether to pursue aggressive treatments or opt for comfort care at home.

The Role of Spirituality in Coping with Aging

Spirituality can offer valuable support for seniors by providing a sense of peace, purpose, and resilience. It helps older adults maintain a positive outlook, which is essential for managing the challenges of aging. Some benefits of spiritual practice include:

Providing Meaning and Purpose: Spirituality can give seniors a reason to keep going, even in difficult times.

- **Accepting Aging**: It can help individuals accept the changes that come with aging, rather than fighting them.

- **Living in the Present**: Spirituality encourages mindfulness and focusing on the present moment, helping to reduce anxiety about the future.

- **Building Social Connections**: Spiritual practices, such as attending religious services or participating in spiritual groups, can foster social connections and reduce loneliness.

- **Supporting Mental and Physical Health**: Spirituality can promote mental well-being by encouraging a positive mind-set, reducing stress, and improving emotional resilience.

- **Encouraging Positivity**: A spiritual outlook can help seniors face challenges with grace and optimism.

- **Offering Comfort**: During times of illness or loss, spirituality can provide emotional comfort and peace.

- **Cultivating Detachment**: Spirituality encourages detachment from material desires, fostering peace and reducing stress.

The Four Ashrams – The Heart of Hinduism

In Hinduism, the life journey is divided into four stages known as the Ashrams. Each stage is meant to develop spiritual qualities and wisdom.

1. **Brahmachari (Student Life):** The first 25 years of life are dedicated to learning, self-discipline, and spiritual growth. This stage focuses on developing virtues like humility, purity, and simplicity.

2. **Grihasta (Household Life):** In this stage, individuals marry, raise a family, and contribute to society. It is the stage where material duties are balanced with spiritual growth, including charitable actions and teaching children spiritual values.

3. **Vanaprashta (Retired Life):** After the children are grown, individuals gradually retire from worldly duties and focus more on spiritual practices, such as meditation, austerities, and pilgrimages.

4. **Sannyasa (Renounced Life):** The final stage involves renouncing worldly possessions and attachments. Individuals dedicate themselves fully to spiritual practice and self-realization, often living a life of simplicity and travel.

SUGGESTIONS for Seniors on Embracing Spirituality and Navigating Aging

Find Meaning and Purpose in Daily Life

Spirituality can provide a renewed sense of purpose. Whether through prayer, meditation, or simply reflecting on life's experiences, seniors can find meaning in each day. Focus on the things that bring you joy and fulfillment— whether that's helping others, engaging in creative activities, or nurturing relationships. By focusing on a higher purpose, you can enhance your overall sense of well-being.

Practice Mindfulness and Acceptance

Aging brings inevitable changes to our bodies and minds. Rather than resisting these changes, spirituality encourages mindfulness and acceptance. Learning to embrace aging as a natural part of life can help reduce stress and anxiety about physical limitations or the fear of mortality. Take time each day to focus on the present moment, whether through quiet reflection, yoga, or simply being mindful of your thoughts and feelings.

Cultivate Social Connections

Spirituality can also foster a sense of community. Participate in spiritual or religious gatherings, whether it's a religious service, study group, or social meeting at a local community centre. These activities provide opportunities to meet new people, build friendships, and reduce feelings of isolation. Volunteering or helping others in need can also provide a sense of belonging and purpose.

Prioritize Mental and Physical Health

Spiritual practices, such as meditation, prayer, or spending time in nature, can help reduce stress and improve emotional health. Additionally, spirituality encourages physical well-being by emphasizing practices like maintaining a balanced diet and engaging in gentle physical activities, such as walking or stretching. Find a balance between nurturing your spiritual and physical health to foster resilience during the aging process.

Focus on Gratitude

Take time each day to reflect on the things you are grateful for. This can include anything from your health, relationships, or simply the beauty of nature. Gratitude can help shift your perspective and foster a more positive outlook, which is essential for coping with the challenges of aging. Keeping a gratitude journal (*Gratitude Journal is a diary of things for which someone is grateful*) can be a simple yet powerful way to focus on the positive aspects of life.

Engage in Acts of Kindness and Service

One of the key aspects of spirituality is contributing to the well-being of others. Whether through charity work, offering advice to younger generations, or helping a neighbour, these acts of kindness can provide a sense of fulfillment and joy. Giving back fosters a deeper connection with others and reinforces the value and purpose you bring to the world.

Reflect on the Four Ashrams of Life

In Hindu philosophy, the journey of life is divided into four stages—*Brahmachari* (Student life), *Grihasta* (Household life), *Vanaprashta* (Retired life), and *Sannyasa* (Renounced life). As seniors, you are likely entering the *Vanaprashta Ashram or Sannyasa Ashram* stage. These stages encourage spiritual growth and detachment from worldly concerns, making room for deeper spiritual exploration. Embrace this stage of life as an opportunity for personal growth, reflection, and focusing on spiritual practices like meditation, pilgrimage, or simply cultivating inner peace.

Accept End-of-Life Thoughts with Grace

As seniors, confronting our own mortality can lead to fear and anxiety. Spirituality can offer comfort during this time by helping you embrace the natural cycle of life. Engage in conversations about your end-of-life wishes, and make peace with the reality of aging. Spirituality can help you approach death with dignity, focusing on the spiritual legacy you wish to leave behind rather than fear or anxiety.

Nurture Your Inner Peace

Spiritual practices can help you find peace, even in the midst of physical or emotional pain. Whether through prayer, meditation, or mindfulness, these practices help reduce stress, promote relaxation, and restore a sense of calm. By prioritizing your inner peace through prayer, meditation, or mindfulness, you can better cope with any challenges that arise and approach aging with more resilience.

Stay Open to Learning

Even in later years, the pursuit of spiritual growth can be fulfilling. Explore different spiritual teachings, engage in philosophical discussions, or read spiritual texts that resonate with you. Keeping your mind engaged and open to new ideas is essential for ongoing growth and maintaining a positive outlook on life.

Conclusion

While aging presents inevitable challenges, spirituality reminds us that we remain valuable and worthy at every stage of life. With the right support, both spiritual and practical, seniors can live fulfilling, peaceful lives, despite the difficulties they may face.

Embracing spirituality can significantly improve the quality of life for seniors, providing comfort, strength, and purpose. By focusing on spiritual practices, building social connections, and cultivating acceptance, seniors can navigate the challenges of aging with greater peace and dignity. Spirituality reminds us that we are not defined by our physical limitations, but by our inner peace, purpose, and connection to the world around us.

Chapter 7

Aging, Quality of Life, and Social Support Available

The quality of life in old age is significantly influenced by social networks and support systems. This chapter will examine the role of family, friends, community, and professional caregivers in enhancing the well-being of older adults. Social isolation is a major risk factor for both mental and physical decline, so fostering strong social connections is essential. I will discuss how staying socially engaged and participating in community activities can improve overall life satisfaction and reduce feelings of loneliness.

Introduction

Aging is a natural process that all individuals experience as they grow older, and it presents unique challenges. In India, as in many other countries, the aging population is increasing due to improvements in healthcare, nutrition, and sanitation. **However, the aging process is often accompanied by physical, emotional, and social challenges that can affect the quality of life.** The issue of aging including the quality of life for senior citizens and the social support systems available to them, is critical in ensuring that older adults lead satisfied and dignified lives. In the chapter I am discussing the key factors related to ageing, the quality of life of elderly people, and the available social support systems in our country.

Aging in India

India has a rapidly aging population. According to the Census 2011, the population of individuals aged 60 and above was about 9% of the total population i.e. about 12 – 13 crore and this number is projected to rise to over 20% by 2050. This demographic shift has significant implications for the country's healthcare systems, economy, and social structures. Many factors contribute to the increase in the elderly population in India, such as improvements in medical care, better living conditions, and advances in technology that prolong life expectancy.

The ageing process is multifaceted, encompassing physical changes, such as reduced mobility and chronic health issues, as well as mental and emotional changes. Older adults may experience isolation, loss of loved ones, and a decline in their ability to participate in social activities. This makes it vital to understand how these factors affect their quality of life.

Quality of Life Among Older Adults

Quality of life refers to the general well-being of individuals, encompassing physical health, mental health, social relationships, and their environment. For elderly people in our country and other developing countries, quality of life is influenced by several factors:

1. **Physical Health**: Chronic illnesses such as arthritis, hypertension, diabetes, and heart disease are prevalent among older adults in India. Access to healthcare services, including preventive care, treatment for diseases, and rehabilitation, plays a crucial role in improving physical well-being. However, the high cost of medical treatment, lack of awareness, and inadequate healthcare infrastructure in rural areas make it difficult for many elderly people to receive timely medical attention.

2. **Mental Health**: Mental health issues, including depression and dementia, are significant concerns for older adults. The social stigma surrounding mental health in India often prevents seniors from seeking the help they need. Furthermore, the lack of specialized mental health services for the elderly aggravate this problem. It is vital to address these mental health challenges to ensure that elderly individuals live with dignity and mental well-being.

3. **Social Involvement**: Social isolation is a major concern for older people in India, especially with the changing family structure. Traditionally, the joint

family system provided support for elderly parents. However, with urbanization and the rise of nuclear families, many elderly individuals are left alone or with limited interaction with family members. This social isolation can lead to feelings of loneliness and depression, further affecting their quality of life.

4. **Financial Security**: Many elderly individuals in India do not have sufficient savings or pensions to support themselves in their later years. In rural areas, where a large proportion of the population resides, there are limited opportunities for older adults to earn an income or find employment. As a result, many elderly individuals rely on family members for financial support, which can lead to dependency and a lack of autonomy.

Social Support Systems in India

Social support for the elderly in India is critical to addressing their needs and enhancing their quality of life. There are several forms of social support, including family, government schemes, and non-governmental organizations (NGOs), each contributing in different ways.

1. **Family Support**: Traditionally, in Indian culture, families play a central role in providing care and support for elderly members. The joint family system, although less common in urban areas today, still remains a vital source of emotional and financial security for older adults. However, the changing family

dynamics and migration of younger generations to urban centers or abroad have created challenges in maintaining this system. This has led to the emergence of elderly people living alone or in retirement homes.

2. **Government Schemes**:   The Indian government has recognized the importance of elderly care and has introduced various policies to ensure the welfare of senior citizens. Some of the key initiatives include:

    - **National Policy on Older Persons (1999)**: This policy aims to ensure that the elderly have access to healthcare, social security, and other essential services.

        The Policy envisages State support to ensure financial and food security, health care, shelter and other needs of older persons, equitable share in development, protection against abuse and exploitation, and availability of services to improve the quality of their lives.

        The Ministry of Social Justice and Empowerment implements a Central Sector Scheme of Integrated Programme for Senior Citizens (IPSrC) under which grants in aid are given for running and maintenance of Senior Citizens Homes (Old Age Homes)/ Continuous Care Homes, Mobile Medicare Units etc. to the Implementing Agencies

    - **Indira Gandhi National Old Age Pension Scheme (IGNOAPS)**: This scheme provides financial assistance to senior citizens below the poverty line.

The scheme "Indira Gandhi National Old Age Pension Scheme (IGNOAPS)" is one of the five sub-schemes of the National Social Assistance Programme (NSAP). Under IGNOAPS, citizens living Below Poverty Line and 60 years or above in age are eligible to apply. A monthly pension is Rs. 200 up to 79 years and Rs. 500 thereafter.

The Government of India, on 15th August 1995, introduced the National Social Assistance Programme (NSAP) as a fully funded Centrally Sponsored Scheme targeting the destitute, defined as any person who has little or no regular means of subsistence from his / her own source of income or through financial support from family members or other sources, to be identified by the States and UTs, with the objective of providing a basic level of financial aid. NSAP is being administered by the Ministry of Rural Development. This program is being implemented in rural areas as well as urban areas.

NSAP represents a significant step towards the fulfillment of the Directive Principles of State Policy enshrined in the Constitution of India which enjoin upon the State to undertake within its means a number of welfare measures. These are intended to secure for the citizen's adequate means of livelihood, raise the standard of living, improve public health, provide free and compulsory education for children, etc.

The NSAP at present includes five sub-schemes as its components -

   a. Indira Gandhi National Old Age Pension Scheme (IGNOAPS)

   b. Indira Gandhi National Widow Pension Scheme (IGNWPS)

   c. Indira Gandhi National Disability Pension Scheme (IGNDPS)

   d. National Family Benefit Scheme (NFBS)

   e. Annapurna Scheme

- **Rashtriya Vayoshri Yojana (2017)**: This initiative aims to provide physical aids and assistive devices to senior citizens to improve their quality of life. However, despite these efforts, there are significant gaps in the effective implementation of these schemes, especially in rural areas. Access to government support remains limited for many elderly people.

3. **Non-Governmental Organizations (NGOs)**: Several NGOs in India focus on the welfare of senior citizens, providing services such as medical care, counselling, recreational activities, and advocacy for elderly rights. These organizations, including Help Age India, Age well Foundation, and others, play an essential role in filling the gaps left by governmental support. They also raise awareness about the challenges faced by older adults and work to ensure their voices are heard in policy discussions.

Help Age India: Set up in 1978, the organisation works for 'the cause and care of disadvantaged older persons to improve their quality of life'. Help Age's motto is 'Fighting isolation, poverty and neglect'. It envisions a society where the elderly has the right to an active, healthy and dignified life.

Age well Foundation: Age well Foundation, India is a not-for-profit organization which has been working for the welfare and empowerment of older persons of India since 1999. Age well interacts with over 25000 older persons on daily basis through its volunteers' nationwide network.

4. **Old Age Homes and Retirement Communities:** As the concept of the nuclear family has become more widespread, retirement homes and old age homes have gained popularity in urban areas. These facilities offer a place for elderly people to live independently or with support, depending on their health needs. While some homes provide a comfortable environment with medical facilities and recreational activities, others struggle with issues like overcrowding, lack of proper healthcare, and insufficient financial resources.

Old-Age Homes: Old-age homes offer the bare minimum facilities. Seniors can expect it to be like an institution where they can spend their sunset years, free from household chores and tasks. But, beyond that, old-age homes lack major facilities.

Key facilities available – rooms for sleeping (mostly dormitories or shared with a couple of other seniors), a common dining hall, a lounge to receive visitors, and common bathrooms. Some of the old age homes in Vadodara are listed below.

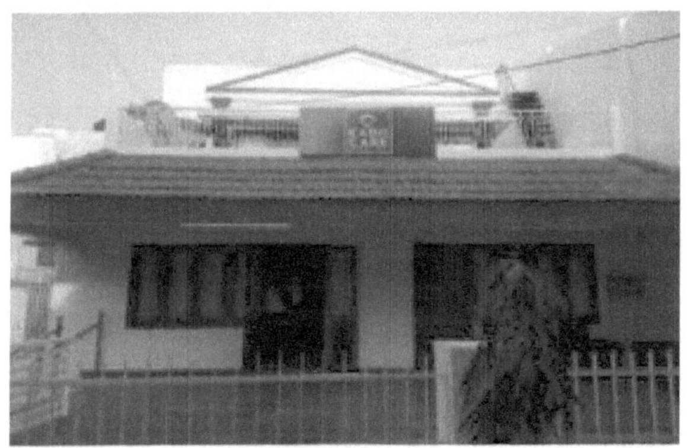

Kadji Care

1. Swarg Community Care

2. Dear Zindagi Senior Care

3. Kadji Care

4. Manya Rehabilitation & Old Age Care

5. Ekta's Carehome Foundation

6. Jalamar Vrudhashram

7. Jatan The Care- Old Age Home

8. Welcare Vatsalya

9. Vadilo No Visamo

10. Amulya Care Home

Cost Of Old Age Homes In Vadodara

The estimated cost of old age homes in Vadodara can vary depending on the level of care and services provided. **Generally, the cost can range from INR 15,000 to INR 50,000 per month per person.** This cost includes basic amenities such as food, accommodation, medical support, and recreational activities. However, additional charges are applied for specialized care, such as dementia care, physiotherapy, and nursing care.

Senior Living Communities

Retirement villages are made up of independent living units known as **senior living homes**. You can consider it as an apartment complex, designed for seniors. So, you can expect all the facilities that you can find in a regular residential apartment complex, with special features to aid seniors.

All apartments are self-contained home units with master bedrooms, guest bedrooms, bathrooms, living rooms, balcony, kitchens, and dining rooms. You are in full control of your apartment, and you have the space to live independently, while the opportunities to mingle and engage with other seniors living in similar residential apartments in the community.

However, since senior living communities are designed for seniors, most apartments contain several accessibility features like gentle slopes, lifts etc., anti-skid floors, chamfered wall edges, easy-reach light switches, night switches in the bedrooms, grab rails in the bathrooms, emergency response system and more. One of such Senior Living Communities has recently opened at Padra, near Vadodara by Banker Group of Hospitals. Details of this given below.

Swajan Bankers Community for luxurious senior care

Swajan offers luxurious amenities, comprehensive healthcare services, and a commitment to sustainability, providing an exceptional living experience ensuring residents safety.

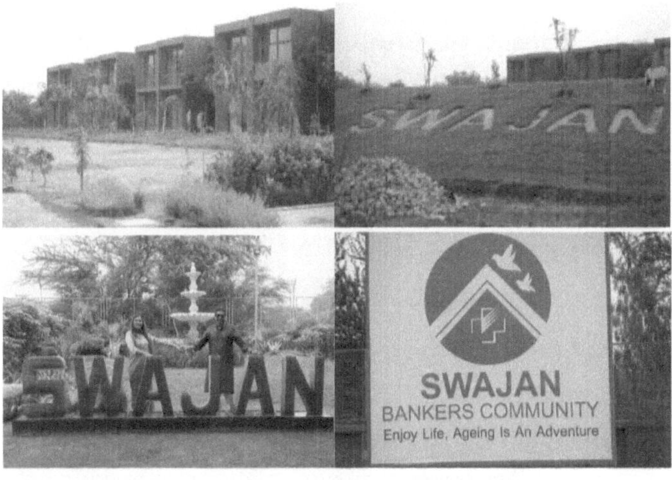

Swajan Community Living has provided a harmonious and fulfilling life for senior residents through exceptional care, vibrant community engagement, and comprehensive healthcare services. They have provided community where seniors can thrive, enjoying a dignified and independent life enriched with activities, companionship, and peace of mind. Here aging is embraced as an adventure and every day is a new opportunity to live life to the fullest. Swajan's approach to senior living ensures that every resident's physical, emotional, and spiritual needs are met. With top-notch healthcare facilities, engaging cultural programs, and a plethora of recreational activities, it creates an environment that promotes well-being and happiness.

Challenges in Elderly Care in India

Despite the growing awareness of elderly issues, several challenges persist. The primary issues include:

- **Inadequate Healthcare Services**: Healthcare services tailored to the elderly are often not available in rural areas, and many seniors cannot afford the high cost of private healthcare. The lack of specialized geriatric care (medical care for older adults) makes it difficult for older adults to receive the attention they need.

- **Cultural Factors**:   The social stigma around aging and mental health, coupled with the traditional expectation that the elderly should live with their families, prevents many seniors from seeking help outside the family.

- **Financial Strain**:   Many elderly people in India face financial insecurity, especially if they are not covered by Government pension schemes or have insufficient personal savings.

- ◆ **Isolation**: The decline of the extended family structure and urban migration has resulted in greater social isolation, leading to feelings of neglect and loneliness among older adults.

Conclusion

Aging in our country presents many challenges for the Government & Society. While there has been progress in addressing the needs of the elderly, significant gaps remain in healthcare, social support, and financial security. The elderly population requires comprehensive attention from the Government, society, and individuals to ensure they live with dignity, independence, and quality of life. It is essential to strengthen social support systems, including the family, Government schemes, and NGOs, to cater to the diverse needs of India's aging population. As the population continues to grow older, it will be crucial to foster an inclusive, supportive environment where older adults can thrive and contribute to society.

Under the above conditions in our country, it is strongly recommended that the seniors of 70 and above must practice Yoga & Meditation under the guidance of trained teachers for better physical and mental health which will help tremendously to cope up with many short comings from the Government and Society sites.

The details of Yoga Exercises, Super Brain Exercises and Meditation are described in detail as Appendix 4, reducing the risk of chronic illnesses and supports overall physical health.

Chapter 8

Medical Aspects: Cardiovascular Diseases, Strokes, Cancer & Other Age-Related Diseases

As people age, the risk of developing certain health conditions increases, leading to a decline in quality of life and sometimes even premature death. Among the most prevalent health problems affecting older adults (around 70) are Cardiovascular Diseases (CVDs), Strokes, Cancer, and a host of other age-related conditions. These health issues, often chronic in nature, require early intervention, lifestyle adjustments, and appropriate care to manage their impact. This chapter explores the common medical conditions in older adults, with a focus on Cardiovascular diseases, strokes, cancer, and other age-related health issues, while offering suggestions for preventing and managing these conditions.

A. Cardiovascular Diseases in Older Adults

Cardiovascular diseases (CVDs), which include a range of conditions, such as Coronary Artery disease, Heart failure, Irregular Heartbeat, and Hypertension, these are among the leading causes or symptom of disease and death in people around 70. **The aging process naturally affects the heart and blood vessels, contributing to the stiffening of arteries, reduced efficiency of the heart, and increase likelihood of plaque build-up, which can obstruct blood flow.**

Factors such as high blood pressure, high cholesterol, smoking, obesity, and a sedentary lifestyle can further increase Cardiovascular risk.

Suggestions for Prevention and Management

Healthy Diet: Eating a heart-healthy diet, rich in fruits, vegetables, whole grains, lean proteins, and low in saturated fats, salt, and sugar, can help lower the cholesterol and blood pressure.

Regular Exercise: Engaging in regular physical activity, such as walking, swimming, or cycling, can improve Cardiovascular health, reduce the risk of heart disease, and maintain a healthy weight.

Monitoring Blood Pressure and Cholesterol: Regular check-ups with a family doctor to monitor blood pressure and cholesterol levels can help early detection of any abnormalities. It is recommended to get all the tests done every six month.

Quit Smoking: Smoking contributes to the hardening of arteries and increases blood pressure and heart rate. If you smoke or use other tobacco products, take help of Doctor to quit this habit of consuming tobacco products.

Manage Stress: Stress will adversely effect your heart. You do your best to reduce stress, if required you can take help of your friends and Doctor for this.

Get Enough Sleep: Quality sleep plays an important role in the healing and repair of your heart and blood vessels. Aim for seven to eight hours sleep per night. If you have difficulty in getting good deep sleep, consult your Doctor about potential solutions, including prescribed sleeping aids.

Medications: For older adults with existing heart conditions, medications like stains, anti hypertensive drugs, and anticoagulants may be prescribed to help manage symptoms and prevent complications.

B. Strokes in Older Adults

A stroke occurs when the blood supply to the brain is interrupted, either due to a blockage (Ischemic stroke) or a rupture of blood vessels (hemorrhagic stroke). The risk of having a stroke increases with age, and older adults are more likely to suffer from its severe consequences. High blood pressure, diabetes, smoking, high cholesterol, and a family history of stroke can all raise the likelihood of having a stroke.

Suggestions for Prevention and Management

Control Risk Factors: Managing high blood pressure, diabetes, and cholesterol through lifestyle changes and medications can significantly reduce stroke risk.

Regular Monitoring: Frequent check-ups, especially for individuals with risk factors, can help in early detection and treatment of underlying issues like Atrial fibrillation or Carotid artery disease.

Physical and Cognitive Rehabilitation: For stroke survivors, rehabilitation programs focusing on Physio therapy, speech therapy, and cognitive rehabilitation are essential for regaining lost functions and improving quality of life.

Healthy Habits: Quitting smoking, reducing alcohol consumption, maintaining a healthy diet, and exercising regularly can lower the overall risk of stroke.

C. Cancer in Older Adults

Cancer is another significant health concern for Older adults. While the incidence of certain cancers, such as breast, prostate, lung, and colorectal cancers, increases with age, early detection and effective treatments have improved survival rates. Factors like genetic, environmental exposures (e.g., smoking, sun exposure), and a weakened immune system can contribute to the higher cancer risk in older adults.

Suggestions for Prevention and Management

Regular Screenings: Early detection through screenings, such as mammograms etc. can lead to earlier treatment with good positive results.

Lifestyle Changes: Avoiding tobacco, and alcohol consumption, maintaining a healthy weight, and exercising regularly can lower the risk of several cancers.

Nutritional Support: A balanced diet rich in Antioxidants (A substance that protects cells from the damage caused by free radicals (unstable molecules made by the process of oxidation during normal metabolism). Free radicals may play a part in cancer, heart disease, stroke, and other diseases of aging) vitamins, and fiber may support the immune system and help reduce cancer risk. Plant-based foods are the best source of antioxidants. These include fruits, vegetables, whole grains, nuts, seeds, herbs and spices, and even cocoa.

Cancer Treatments and Palliative Care: For individuals diagnosed with cancer, a combination of surgery, chemotherapy, radiation therapy can be used depending on the type and stage of cancer. In advanced stages, medical treatment and Palliative care (a type of medical care that helps people with serious illnesses live a better quality of life) can help to manage symptoms and improve quality of life. For cancer, nutritional support is vital for maintaining strength during treatment.

Other Common Age-Related Diseases

In addition to cardiovascular diseases, strokes, and cancer, older adults are also vulnerable to a variety of other conditions, such as issues with bones, joints and muscles, digestive system, your bladder and urinary track, eyes and ears, memory and thinking capabilities, diabetes, arthritis, osteoporosis, cognitive decline (including Alzheimer's disease and other dementia), and respiratory diseases like Chronic Obstructive Pulmonary Disease (COPD). These conditions, often intertwined with one another, can result in diminished functionality and independence, impacting an individual's overall well-being.

i. **Bones, joints and muscles**

With age, bones tend to shrink in size and density. This weakens them. Age-related bone changes also might cause reduction in size. Muscles tend to lose strength and flexibility and this in turn can effect coordination, stability and balance. These changes raise the risk of falls and fractures.

To maintain healthy bones, joints and muscles, it is essential to consume sufficient calcium, vitamin - D, engage in regular exercise, and avoid substances like tobacco, excessive alcohol etc.

ii. **Digestive System**

Age-related structural changes in the large intestine can result in constipation in seniors, not drinking enough fluids, low fiber diet etc., medications such as

Diuretics and Iron supplements and certain medical conditions.

To prevent constipation, consume a healthy diet high in fiber, drink plenty of water and other fluids. Regular physical activity in your daily routine will help to prevent constipation. Lastly do not ignore the urge to have a bowel movement. Holding in a bowel for too long can cause constipation.

iii. Bladder and Urinary Tract:

As you age, your bladder may become less elastic resulting in the need to urinate more often. Weakening bladder muscles and pelvic floor muscles may make it difficult for you to emptying the bladder completely or cause you to lose bladder control (urinary incontinence). In men, an enlarged or inflamed prostate also can cause difficult emptying the bladder and incontinence.

To promote bladder and urinary tract, consider the following tips:

- Go to the toilet regularly. Consider urinating on a regular schedule, such as every hour. Slowly, extend the amount of time between your toilet trips.

- Maintain a healthy weight. If you're overweight, lose excess pounds.

- Don't smoke. If you smoke or use other tobacco product, ask your Doctor to help you quit.

- Do Kegel exercises. To exercise your pelvic floor muscles (Kegel exercises), squeeze the muscles you would use to stop passing gas. **Take help of Yoga Teacher or Physiotherapist.**

iv. Eyes and Ears:

During aging you may experience difficulty focusing on near objects, increase sensitivity to glare, and difficulty adopting to changes in light. Aging can also effect the eye's lens leading to cataracts, which require attention from an ophthalmologist.

Similarly for poor hearing, consult ENT specialist and use hearing Aid.

v. Memory and Thinking Skills:

As the brain ages, some individuals may experience minor effects on memory and cognitive functions (thinking skills). For instance, healthy older adults might forget familiar names or words, or multitask effectively.

Cognitive health can be maintained by engaging in regular physical activity in your daily routine, eat a healthy diet, staying mentally active, staying socially engaged, Quitting smoking and early treatment for any cardiovascular issues (diseases) as and when noticed. No delay.

Suggestions for Prevention and Management

Regular Health Check-ups: Regular visits to healthcare providers for managing chronic conditions like diabetes, arthritis, and respiratory diseases can prevent complications and manage symptoms effectively. Follow your Doctor's advice about glasses, contact lenses, hearing aids, using pace-maker and other corrective devices.

Bone Health: Weight-bearing exercises, adequate calcium and vitamin D intake, and medications for osteoporosis can help reduce the risk of fractures.

Cognitive Health: Keeping the brain active through mental exercises, social engagement, and healthy lifestyle choices can help delay or prevent cognitive decline.

Physical Therapy: For conditions like arthritis and osteoporosis, physical therapy can improve mobility, reduce pain, and enhance overall physical function.

Conclusion

Due to lifestyle factors and genetics, Cardiovascular diseases, strokes, cancer, and other age-related conditions are common among older adults. However, many of these conditions are preventable or manageable with early detection, proper treatment, and healthy lifestyle choices. By adopting preventive measures such as a balanced diet, regular exercise, routine health screenings, and managing chronic conditions, older adults can significantly improve their health and enjoy a better quality of life. **The key to healthy aging lies in a proactive and holistic approach to healthcare that emphasizes prevention, treatment, and ongoing care.**

Chapter 9

Real Life Examples

In this chapter, we share real-life stories of people in our circle of friends, relatives, and neighbour who are around 70 years old or older. These examples show different ways people deal with the challenges of aging.

This case is of Shri Girish Vithal & His Family: Example of Positive Attitude, Calmness and Willingness

I would like to demonstrate with a live example how the attitude and willingness of a person can overcome the genetic influence on him/her.

I have a friend named Shri Girish Kumar Vithal who is born in a middle class joint family in 1955. He has 3 sisters and one brother, all grown in a joint family. All of them are graduate but because of his willingness and dedication, Shri Vithal completed his post-graduation in Chemistry and was selected as Scientific Officer in the prestigious scientific research organization viz. Bhabha Atomic Research Centre known popularly as BARC.

At an early age of 22 years, the financial responsibility of the entire joint family came on his shoulders as his father passed away at the age of 51 years. That time his one of the two elder sisters was married while one younger sister and brother were studying. Being foresighted, he decided that he will get married only after arranging the marriage of his elder as well as younger sister.

In the meantime, Shri Vithal took transfer from Mumbai to Kota so that he can better take care of his mother and other family members, residing at Delhi. He finally got married at the age of 29 years in 1984. He also got the professional responsibility as Head of Process Chemistry and Analytical Laboratory in Heavy Water Plant, Kota, an industrial unit of Department of Atomic Energy, which is situated 60 km away from Kota. In 1993, his wife who was a lecturer in junior college had developed bipolar disorder. **He very boldly accepted the challenge of keeping her wife motivated to face the disease and continue her teaching.** He continued to manage and balance his professional responsibility and visiting Doctors at Kota City with his wife as and when required. I and my other family members **never saw him perturbed or unhappy. This could be possible because of his positive attitude, will power as well as willingness to win over the problems.**

Subsequently, Vithal family adopted a baby as a part of their family. Mrs Vithal was continuously under treatment as she continued to have few episodes of bipolar attacks. His daughter was growing and was very intelligent and active. In 2003, Mr Vithal was promoted to Manager Process Chemistry and Quality Control and was transferred to the Head office at Mumbai. Everything was going well when one day in 2007, **Doctor informed him that his daughter, Mahima, who was in 9th class was suffering from INCURABLE Auto Immune Disorder disease called SLE** Systemic Lupus Erethematosus - An inflammatory disease caused when the immune system attacks its own tissues. Doctor informed that Mahima has to be continuously on Steroids but still it is not sure how long Lupus will remain dormant. This was the most shocking period of Shri Vithal family. Within a month, Mr Vithal composed himself and with his positive attitude encouraged the entire family and relatives to face the reality and provided Mahima whatever best treatment is available. He boosted the will power of his daughter and wife not to get depressed and believe in themselves to face the situation and pray to God to give them strength for the same. Slowly emotional situation becoming normal and treatment with frequent follow ups continued.

Mahima completed her 10th with 92%, 12th with 93% and BE Electrical with 74% even though she was in between to be taken to hospitals for various follow ups/ hospital admission. She was determined to achieve her goals irrespective of her uncertainty in the health. She wanted to do MBA but on Mr Vithal's advice, she first took her Job as Engineer in R&D Group of Schneider Electric

Bangluru for 2 years in 2015 when Mr Vithal retired and settled in Vadodara.

Afterwards when Mahima resigned in 2017 and came to Vadodara for MBA preparation, within a month Lupus got active and attacked her kidneys and within a month she was on tri-weekly Dialysis (Online 4 hours technique to purify body blood). That was another big jolt on Vithal family. Again his Will Power did not allow him to be perturbed from his aim to do the best for her daughter.

Mahima needed one kidney transplant from a healthy family member so that torturous dialysis procedure of 4 hours thrice a week for life long can be stopped. Mr Vithal got to know from Sonography that he has only 1 matured kidney by birth and his wife has healthy kidneys but she has different Blood Group than Mahima. Initially his brother assured him that he or his wife will donate his/her kidney as both of them have same blood group as Mahima, but when Mahima was made ready for transplant, both of his brother and bhabhi took U turn. Again and again Destiny was putting the family to Acid Tests. This time Mrs Vithal proved her commitment and boldness by donating her kidney in 2018. After kidney transplant, Mahima proved her commitment by getting 90th rank in MBA entrance test conducted by Gujarat State in 2019. Finally Mahima got 11th rank in MBA all courses at Navrachna University, Vadodara in 2021. In between, Mahima ranked 5th in Vadodara District and 8th in Gujarat State in an open "Public Speaking Competition" organised by Times of India Group.

In 2021, during COVID-19, Mahima got infected and her working kidney got rejected leading to 15 days isolation with again starting of tri-weekly dialysis. This was a bigger shock for the parents but very big shock for Mahima. She started getting depressed and Mrs Vithal's bipolar attacks also getting increased. During all these incidents, Mr Vithal's Friends (5 colleagues for 40 years and all staying together in the same housing Society at Vadodara) were always available for every kind of moral and physical support but there was hardly any help available from relatives except disturbing the family through almost daily telephoning and asking about Mahima regularly. This time Mr Vithal was really put into a corner. He was to simultaneously look after Mahima and Mrs Vithal. He was either to stay 24*7 with Mahima when she got admitted in hospital or during dialysis and at the same time coordinating through video calls with friends to take care of Mrs Vithal and her regular doses of various medicines. **I saw the dedication, coolness and patience with which Mr Vithal was accepting every situation and managing everyone along with family's day to day responsibility.**

Even with all out efforts and the best possible treatment, Mahima passed away on 26th May 2022 giving the biggest trauma to the parents. That was the only time I saw Mr Vithal breaking down. This time he took almost 4 months to compose himself and brought his Will Power back to accept the fact of Mahima leaving them. But Mrs Vithal's health started deteriorating and was to be admitted quite frequently for bipolar episodes. Mr Vithal is again taking care of her with full dedication and coolness.

Conclusion

In conclusion, the life of Shri Girish Kumar Vithal stands as a testament to the remarkable will power and positive attitude in overcoming life's immense challenges. His journey, marked by personal and professional achievements, was not without his share of several hardships. Despite the immense problems faced by his family, including the health struggles of both his wife and daughter, Shri Vithal's unwavering determination, foresight, and resilience allowed him to not only maintain composure but also inspire those around him to remain strong in the face of adversity. His ability to remain calm, take bold decisions, and navigate through life's difficulties with grace and perseverance highlights the incredible impact of a positive mind-set. Through his experiences, we learn that while life may present numerous challenges which are almost impossible to overcome, **it is ultimately one's will power, attitude, and determination that shape our ability to overcome them.**

A Tribute to Author's Dadaji:
Legacy of Determination and Inner Strength

This is a live example of inner Strength, Spiritualism, Determination, Discipline and Family support. My paternal grandfather, the late Shri Rala Ramji, was a living example of internal strength, disciplined living, and unwavering spiritualism. Born and raised in Lyallpur, West Pakistan, he led a prosperous life through wholesale grain trading and money lending. His success and hard work ethic formed the foundation of a stable and happy family, with three sons and three daughters who gave lot of respect to him. But it was during an unprecedented phase of his life that the true depth of his character and determination became evident.

In 1938, at the age of 75, my Dadaji lost his eyesight, a devastating blow for any individual. Yet, even with this immense personal challenge, he did not loss his confidence and determination. He continued to be a pillar of support and guidance to his family. His very brave and determined spirit remained unbroken as he adjusted to life without sight, demonstrating resilience that left a profound impact on all who knew him.

The most defining test of his strength came during the troubled period of the Partition of India in 1947. Forced to leave his home in the face of violence and uncertainty, he travelled with his family from the refugee camp in Pakistan to the Indian side and finally to Delhi. Despite being 75 years old and blind, Dadaji faced these trials with an unshakable will. He journeyed by foot, bus, and train, moving through the chaos with remarkable grace. Even in his senior years, he remained calm and composed offering stability and wisdom to his loved ones in the midst of displacement and hardship.

Beyond his physical resilience, Dadaji's disciplined lifestyle stood out. He maintained a strict routine, waking up at 5 AM and retiring at 9 PM every day. With the help of my grandmother, Dadi, he managed to take care of his personal needs, and each morning, a grandchild would accompany him to the local temple. His faith was his constant companion, and he would spend time in prayer and reflection, listening to *Bhajans* and *Aartis*. This daily ritual not only exemplified his devotion but also set an example for the younger generation in the family, showing the importance of maintaining one's health, spiritual practices, and inner peace.

What truly sets Dadaji apart, though, is the manner in which he led his life. Despite the challenges of blindness and age, he never displayed anger or frustration. He interacted with everyone around him in a calm and composed manner, always adjusting to the needs of others and ensuring that he never became a burden. His humility, patience, and compassion created an atmosphere of love and respect within the family.

Even in his final years, Dadaji's spirit remained strong. He passed away in 1962 at the age of 99, leaving behind a legacy of hard work, resilience, and love. His teachings, especially his deep faith in *Bhagwan*, and his ability to stay disciplined and positive in the face of adversity, continue to inspire us to this day. His life was a testament to the power of internal strength, and his example of determination and willpower remains a guiding light for all who had the privilege to know him. In fact my daily routine and disciplined life style is because of my Dadaji's teachings.

Conclusion

Dadaji's story is not just one of personal triumph but a living example of how we should face life's challenges. His life, full of unwavering spiritualism, determination, and discipline, continues to be inspiration of hope and inspiration for our entire family. His legacy of strength, grace, and devotion to family and faith lives on in all of us.

Author's Own Case:
Example of Positivity, Sensitivity, Speed & Self Confidence

I came to India at the age of 5 years in 1947 from Pakistan after the partition of India with my parents. My parents had to struggle to settle as Refugee and I was sent to my *Nanaji* place where I studied till 11th class. Then I came back to my parents and completed my B.Sc. My ambition was to study abroad for higher education. I am grateful to my grandparents and parents, who instilled discipline and a positive attitude. Further I put my hard work to achieve my ambition and got Ph.D. Chemical Engineering from United Kingdom. All the subsequent details are documented in my Autobiography titled " Ek Refugee Scientist" published in 2024.

My experiences exemplify the power of **signaling**, **alertness**, **confidence**, and **willpower** in overcoming life-threatening health challenges like heart attacks and strokes. My journey showcases how positive thinking, attentiveness to health, and self-confidence can be crucial for overcoming such critical situations. Let's break down these aspects to provide a detailed understanding of how each contributed to my survival and recovery.

Signaling/Alertness: Recognizing and Responding to Warning Signs

In my case, the key of managing my Cardiovascular health was my ability to recognise **the warning signs** early on. In 1977, after my short fainting spell, the first signal came in the form of a **minor heart attack**. This initial incident served as a **nature's warning**—a call of action to prioritise my health. I recognised the importance of listening to my body and heeding these signs, a vital skill for anyone facing a heart attack or stroke. Early identification of symptoms is crucial for timely intervention and can greatly improve survival rates.

Later, in 2008, when I faced breathing difficulties during a morning walk in NIT, Hamirpur, Himachal Pradesh, I quickly recognised that these were warning signs of a Cardiovascular issue. My **sensitivity to my body's signals** enabled me to take proactive measures. I did not ignore these signs, instead made the decision to seek medical advice and promptly returned home for further evaluation. **This ability to act on subtle warning signs is an example of how alertness can save lives.**

I carefully assessed my breathing difficulties and, without hesitation, shared my concerns with my friends and medical professional, Prof. Jairal. This allowed them to make an informed decision to return to Jalandhar for further diagnosis. Additionally, when I felt the same symptoms in 2019 while taking stairs in Baroda, my awareness of my body's state prompted me to immediately seek medical evaluation.

My ongoing vigilance in monitoring these symptoms—even in seemingly normal activities—was the key. It wasn't just about feeling unwell, but **being mentally attuned to the fact that something could be wrong**, which propelled me to take immediate action, including seeking professional care.

Confidence: Belief in Timely Medical Intervention

Confidence is not just about mental strength but also about **trusting the process** and professionals in times of crisis. In my case, my confidence in our medical team, especially during crucial procedures, was a cornerstone of my recovery. When I was diagnosed with 90% blockage in my arteries, I trusted Doctors' advice and opted for immediate stenting instead of delaying the procedure, even when there was no emergency.

This timely decision, made with confidence in the expertise of my medical team, helped prevent further complications. Similarly, in 2019, when I experienced another heart attack, my unwavering confidence in the quick response of Dr. Parul Banker and the hospital team enabled me to remain calm and focused on my recovery, despite the complex nature of my condition. **This belief in swift and appropriate medical intervention was instrumental in overcoming the crisis.**

Willpower: Determination to Overcome the Crisis

Throughout these episodes, I displayed an incredible willpower—a mental resolve to keep fighting and maintain optimism, even in the face of life-threatening health challenges. Following my heart attack in 2019, despite the seriousness of my condition, I remained determined to survive, telling myself daily that I would be cured. This mental strength, repeated in daily affirmations, was a critical factor in my recovery.

Additionally, after experiencing further health setbacks, my determination to continue the treatment and my belief in the possibility of recovery remained unshaken. Willpower kept me going, and my ongoing positive affirmation helped me stay mentally strong throughout.

Speed: Swift Action during Critical Moments

The speed at which I responded to my health episodes highlights the importance of quick thinking during emergencies. Whether it was the rapid decision to seek medical help after my fainting spell in 1977 or my immediate response to a potential blockage in 2008 and 2019, my swift actions ensured that I received timely medical intervention. For instance, after my second heart attack in 2019, the immediate contact with Dr. Parul Banker and the quick organization of ICU care were pivotal in ensuring that I received prompt attention.

In an emergency like a heart attack or stroke, every second counts. My ability to quickly recognize the gravity of the situation and make prompt decisions saved my life multiple times.

Conclusion

In conclusion, my life and experiences serve as a powerful example of how positivity, sensitivity, speed, self-confidence, and willpower can make a significant difference in overcoming life-threatening health challenges. My ability to recognize early warning signs, stay alert to symptoms, trust in medical professionals, and act swiftly in critical moments has been central to my survival and recovery. Moreover, my unshakable willpower and positive mindset have empowered me to navigate multiple health crises with resilience. My journey underscores the importance of a proactive and confident approach to health, inspiring others to prioritize self-awareness, timely intervention, and determination in the face of adversity.

The Case of Dr. (Mrs.) Kiran Shingari: Example of Family Support

This narrative is about my wife, Dr. Mrs. Kiran Shingari. She earned her Ph.D. in Electronics at the age of 25 from IIT, Banaras Hindu University, and we have now been happily married for over 53 years. Our marriage has been a source of mutual support and joy for more than five decades.

After our marriage in 1972, Kiran joined my company and worked alongside me for 13 years, until 1985. In 1986, we mutually decided that she would leave her professional career to focus on raising our two children, Gaurav and Amar, and managing our home. Before this, Kiran had also resigned from her position as a lecturer at Women's College, BHU, to prioritize family life.

For many years, she dedicated herself wholeheartedly to our home, ensuring that our children were well-educated, happy, and supported. Kiran efficiently managed every aspect of household life, from day-to-day chores to creating a nurturing environment for our family. She did all of this with immense energy and dedication until she turned 60.

However, as time passed, I began to notice certain changes in Kiran. Her once-boundless energy began to decline, and she frequently remarked that "old age is catching up with us." While I always reassured her that age is just a number, and I refused to see myself as old, it was clear that things were changing. Kiran, now 80 years old, has faced physical challenges, including undergoing both knee replacements in 2016 and 2017, marking the beginning of her health issues. Alongside this, there were noticeable shifts in her behaviour and attitude:

- **Memory Issues**: She began to struggle with short-term memory loss.

- **Slower Physical Activity**: Her physical movements and energy levels slowed down.

- **Decreased Walking Speed:** She started walking more slowly and tried to avoid to go out.

- **Slower Thought Processes:** Her thinking became less sharp and she started taking more time in decision making.

- **Increased Indoor Time:** She spent a lot of time with domestic help, watching TV, and using her mobile phone.

- **Shrinking Social Circle:** Her social interactions became limited to a small circle of relatives.

- **Increased Nervousness:** She became nervous and anxious than usual for an unplanned event.

I also began to observe noticeable behavioral changes that mirrored those of her parents. In the mornings, she exhibited traits similar to her father, while in the afternoons, she seemed to take on characteristics of her mother. On certain occasions, Kiran would appear more like the vibrant, younger version of herself, which reminded me of the woman I married all those years ago. Though I mentioned these changes to her, she neither confirmed nor denied them.

I strongly believe that genetics plays a significant role in shaping a person's behaviour, but environmental factors and life experiences also contribute equally to changes in personality and outlook.

These changes in Kiran's health and behaviour were not only noticed by me but by other members of our family, including Gaurav, Amar, Lovely, and Poonam. Together, we decided to take collective action to support her:

- **Creating a Positive Environment**: We made sure that Kiran was always surrounded by positive energy and that all family members maintained a supportive attitude toward her. We subtly encouraged her to adopt a more optimistic outlook.

- **Fostering Conversations with Grandchildren**: We encouraged her to share her experiences of University life, teaching at college, and working in our family business with the grandchildren. This not only gave her a sense of purpose but also strengthened family bonds.

- **Spiritual Practices**: We started a family ritual of going to our temple and performing joint Pooja every evening at 7 PM. To make it easier for her to participate, we purchased large-print versions of the *Ramayana* and *Geeta*, so she could read along during Pooja. Additionally, I began practicing Yoga and Meditation, and then sharing the mental and physical benefits I felt from these practices.

- **Mental Stimulation**: Amar bought her a book of puzzles to engage her mind and improve concentration.

- **Spiritual Discussions**: We introduced discussions on spirituality during our evening tea, explaining how spirituality could provide her with emotional strength and mental clarity. These discussions became a source of comfort and support for all of us.

- **Encouraging Social Interactions**: We ensured that Kiran attended family and friends' gatherings at home, which encouraged her social interactions and helped her stay connected to the world outside our home.

Through these efforts, we were able to restore much of Kiran's confidence and improve her emotional well-being. Today, I am happy to report that she has made a remarkable recovery. Her confidence has grown, and she is now actively participating in social events and engaging with our grandchildren, guests, and even our domestic help. She has become more independent, occasionally going for shopping with the driver to handle household purchases.

One member of the family accompanies her during these outings to ensure her safety, as we wanted to prevent any falls, which had become more frequent in the past. To further ensure her comfort and safety, we made several modifications in our bathrooms to prevent accidents.

This journey has been a testament to the importance of family support, especially from the head of the family, in restoring confidence, health, and happiness in our senior family members. Through our collective efforts, we've seen Dr. Kiran Shingari, my wife is regaining much of her former vitality and spirit.

We are deeply grateful for the transformation we have witnessed in her, and we hope our example will serve as a reminder to others for the power of family support and the positive impact it can have on a loved one's well-being.

Conclusion

The narrative of Dr. (Mrs.) Kiran Shingari highlights the critical importance of family support in maintaining well-being, particularly as we age. Through collective family efforts—ranging from emotional encouragement and engaging activities to physical and spiritual practices—the Shingari family successfully restored Kiran's confidence and health. Their proactive approach serves as a powerful example of how a positive and supportive environment can significantly impact the recovery and vitality of a senior family member. The experience reinforces the necessity of vigilance and timely action when it comes to health, demonstrating that attentive care, both physical and emotional, can greatly enhance quality of life.

Additionally, the story emphasizes the significance of maintaining a strong family bond, engaging in positive conversations, and offering practical support to ensure the elderly feel connected and valued. The recovery of Dr. Kiran Shingari stands as a testament to the power of love, care, and support within a family, encouraging others to recognize the importance of these elements in fostering resilience and promoting overall well-being.

Chapter 10

Aging Gracefully

(Essential Health Strategies for Seniors)

As we age, the importance of maintaining a balanced and sustainable lifestyle becomes even more critical. Apart from taking precautions related to major diseases like Cardio Vascular Disease, Cancer etc. one shall also be concerned about day to day issues related to digestion, vision, hearing and tendency to fall. This chapter explores some crucial aspects of senior's health.

1. **Caring Your bones, joints and muscles**

    With age, bones tend to shrink in size and density. This weakens them. Muscles tend to lose strength, endurance and flexibility. That in turn can affect coordination, stability and balance. These changes raise the risk of falls. Falling with weaker bones makes it more likely that you could break a bone. This is the worst situation for Senior Adults as some of the broken joints can't be repaired/ replaced around 75-80 and person becomes immobile/bed ridden and always needs a helping hand. Bed ridden for a long time also leads to bedsores aggravating further difficulties for the individual as well as family members. I would like to mention here about 90 years old grandmother of my friend Mr Girish Kumar Vithal who was Chief Chemist in Heavy Water Plant Kota during 1995. I was seeing her very active and healthy till 85 years of age when she fell in the bathroom and broke her hip joint. She became bed ridden and slowly started forgetting about her present and remembering the past incidents. Over the years she forgot to recognize her daughters though her diet and all pathological parameters were very much normal. Subsequently she had bedsores and even after best possible treatment and Care, she passed away at the age of 92. So just because of falling down in bathroom, her last 5 years were very difficult and same was for the entire family.

To help bones, joints and muscles stay healthy

- Get enough calcium. Adults should aim to get at least 1,000 milligrams (mg) of calcium a day. Women age 51 and older, and men 71 and older should aim to get 1,200 mg a day. You can get calcium from foods such as Dairy products, Broccoli, Drumstick etc. If you find it hard to get enough calcium from your diet, ask your Doctor about calcium supplements.

- Get enough Vitamin D. Adults up to age 70 should aim to get 600 International units (IU) of

Vitamin D a day. Adults older than 70 should aim to get 800 IU a day. Sources of Vitamin D include Direct Sunlight, eggs, Vitamin D-fortified milk and Vitamin D supplements.

- Weight-bearing exercises can help you build strong bones and slow bone loss like slow walking for senior citizens while jogging, tennis, climbing stairs and weight training for young ones.

- Smoking tobacco and drinking alcohol can lessen bone mass and raise the risk of fractures. Quit smoking. Also quit alcohol as it can raise the risk of serious injuries from falls and car accidents.

2. **Caring your Digestive system**

Age-related structural changes in the large intestine can result in more constipation in older adults. Other contributing factors include a lack of exercise, not drinking enough fluids and a low-fibre diet. Medications, such as diuretics and iron supplements, and certain medical conditions, such as diabetes, also might contribute to constipation.

To prevent constipation

- Eat a healthy diet. Make sure your diet includes high-fiber foods, such as fruits, vegetables and whole grains. Limit high-fat meats, dairy products and sweets, which might cause constipation. Drink plenty of water and other fluids.

- Regular physical activity can help prevent constipation.

- Holding in a Bowel movement for too long can cause constipation.

3. **Bladder and Urinary tract**

Your bladder may become less elastic as you age, resulting in the need to urinate more often. Weakening of bladder muscles and pelvic floor muscles may make it difficult for you to empty your bladder completely or cause you to lose bladder control (urinary Incontinence). In men, an enlarged or inflamed prostate also can cause difficult emptying the bladder and Incontinence (a person leaks urine by accident).

Incontinence is due to active bladder (Loss of bladder control), varying from a slight loss of urine after sneezing, coughing or laughing to complete inability to control urination.

Other factors that contribute to Incontinence include being overweight, nerve damage from diabetes, certain medications, and Caffeine or Alcohol consumption.

To promote bladder and urinary tract health:

Go to the toilet regularly. Consider urinating on a

- regular schedule, such as every hour. Slowly, extend the amount of time between your toilet trips.

- If you're overweight, lose excess pounds.

- Don't smoke.

- Do Kegel exercises. To exercise your pelvic floor muscles (Kegel exercises), squeeze the muscles you would use to stop passing gas. Try it for 3 seconds at a time, and then relax for a count of 3. Work up to doing the exercise 10 to 15 times in a row, at least 3 times a day.

- Caffeine, Acidic foods, Alcohol and Carbonated beverages can make incontinence worse.

- Eat more fibre and take other steps to avoid constipation, which otherwise can worsen Incontinence.

4. Memory and thinking skills

Your brain undergoes changes as you age that may have minor effects on your memory or thinking skills. For example, **Healthy older adults might forget familiar names or words, or they may find it more difficult to multitask.**

Promote cognitive health by taking the following steps:

Physical activity increases blood flow to your whole body, including your brain. Studies suggest regular exercise is associated with better brain function and reduces stress and depression — factors that affect memory.

- A Heart-healthy Diet may benefit your brain. Focus on fruits, vegetables and whole grains. Choose low-fat protein sources, such as fish, lean meat and skinless poultry. Alcohol can lead to confusion and memory loss.

- Stay mentally active. It may help sustain your memory and thinking skills. You can read, play word games, take up a new hobby, take classes, or learn to play an instrument.

- Social interaction helps ward off depression and stress, which can contribute to memory loss. You might volunteer at a local school or non-profit organization, spend time with family and friends, or attend social events.

- Follow your Doctor's recommendations to manage Cardiovascular risk factors — high blood pressure, high cholesterol and diabetes — that may increase the risk of cognitive decline.

- Quit smoking to help your cognitive health.

5. **Teeth, Eyes and Ears**

With age, you might have difficulty in chewing, focusing on objects and hearing. Teeth become brittle. **You might become more sensitive to glare and have trouble adapting to different levels of light.** Aging also can affect your eye's lens, causing clouded vision (Cataracts).

You might have difficulty hearing High frequencies or following a conversation in a crowded room.

To promote teeth, eye and ear health:

- Schedule regular check-ups. Follow your Doctor's advice about dentures/ implant teeth, glasses/ contact lenses, hearing aids and other corrective devices.

- Wear Sunglasses or a wide-brimmed hat when you're outdoors, and use earplugs when you're around loud machinery or other loud noises.

For seniors, particularly those around 70 years of age, everyday decisions about exercise, diet, work, and rest can significantly impact overall health and quality of life. The following habits will always be useful to keep them more healthy:

1. **Proper Personal Hygiene**

    A lack of good personal hygiene can lead to various issues for seniors. Proper elderly personal hygiene can reduce the risk of hygiene-related diseases and conditions such as:

    Chronic diarrhoea

    Head lice

    Ringworm

    Skin infections

    Tooth decay and gum disease

    Reduced immune system function in seniors can make these conditions a more serious threat to physical health. Not only does proper hygiene help protect against these illnesses, but it can also contribute to overall health for people with chronic conditions like Type 2 diabetes.

Regular hand washing and other grooming tasks can lead to fewer incidents of colds and flu, increasing the importance of personal hygiene for older people with impaired immune systems.

Elderly hygiene also impacts how older people interact with others around them. A consistent hygiene routine makes a person less likely to develop bad breath and body odour.

Conversely, poor elderly personal hygiene can increase the risk of isolation, contributing to depression and anxiety in seniors.

Personal hygiene includes

Gently cleaning your body every day preferably with warm water paying special attention to areas that sweat and smell.

Washing your hands with soap and water after visiting outside, handling pets etc.

Brushing and flossing your teeth twice a day.

Covering your mouth and nose with a Face mask to prevent dust and pollutants in the air.

2. **Overdoing Physiotherapy Exercises**

Physiotherapy (PT) treatment helps to restore movement and function during injury, illness, all types of pains and aches including back pain, shoulder pain, neck pain, bone pain muscular pain and soft tissues etc. It helps to treat orthopaedics, neurological and heart related diseases.

PT uses various methods such as massages, heat treatment therapy, electro therapy etc. It improves strength, flexibility and mobility by reducing or eliminating above mentioned issues. In many cases physiotherapy is must after operations etc.

Physiotherapy is a valuable tool for maintaining mobility and managing chronic conditions. However, overdoing exercises beyond what is recommended by a physiotherapist or Doctor can lead to adverse outcomes. Excessive strain on joints, muscles, or pre-existing injuries can cause inflammation, delayed healing, or even new injuries. Seniors should adhere strictly to the prescribed routines, focusing on proper technique and gradual progression. Consulting a physiotherapist regularly and listening to one's body are essential steps to avoid overexertion.

3. **Overeating and Dietary Considerations**

There are many reasons for natural decline of appetite as we age, including aging itself, the impact of medications, psychological impacts, changes in senses like smell, taste etc. Also our activity has reduced considerably due to retirement and other reasons and hence our requirement for the calories required is less and we should accordingly plan our balanced diet.

There is a tendency that we always compare our old age diet with the younger days and try to overeat than we require at this age. Overeating can lead to weight gain, increased strain on the heart and joints, and a higher risk of conditions like diabetes and hypertension. Seniors must follow age-appropriate dietary plans that emphasize portion control, fibre-rich foods, lean proteins, healthy fats, and adequate hydration. Consulting a dietitian for personalized recommendations can ensure that nutritional needs are met without overloading the digestive system.

4. **Coping with Extreme Weather Conditions**

The extreme weather, such as temperatures above 50°C or around 1°C, pose significant risks to senior health. High heat can lead to dehydration, heatstroke, and cardiovascular stress is very dangerous for seniors above 70. High heat can lead to dehydration, heatstroke, and cardiovascular stress is very dangerous for seniors above 70 than the younger people. Hot weather can cause difficulty in the body's ability to regulate its temperature. This can be challenging as seniors cannot adjust to sudden temperature changes. Heat related illnesses are sudden dizziness, fainting if you are heart patient and taking beta blockers. The other effects of heat are heat cramps, heat oedema, skin irritation from heavy sweating, heat exhaustion and heat strokes.

Exposure to very cold weather around 1 Deg. C to 5 Deg. C will weaken immune system making it easier for common cold and flu viruses to affect and attack. Also very cold weather reduces blood circulation which can hinder the body's ability to fight off infection. Also heart has to work very hard to maintain body's temperature. Very cold weather is dangerous for heart patients. If immunity is low frost bites can cause damage to body tissues.

For older seniors above 70 years longer exposure to severe cold weather increases the risk of hypothermia, respiratory diseases, joint stiffness, heart attack, strokes and depression etc. Arthritis which is very common at this age will also worsen.

Seniors should take appropriate precautions, such as staying indoors during extreme weather, using heating, dressing in multi layers during cold spells, and maintaining hydration. Regular health checks during such times can prevent complications.

5. **The Risks of Overworking After 75 Years**

While staying active and engaged is beneficial for mental and physical health, overworking at advanced ages can lead to fatigue, stress, and worsening of existing health conditions. Seniors should focus on activities that bring joy and fulfillment without causing physical or mental strain. Setting realistic goals, incorporating regular breaks, and seeking help when necessary are essential practices. Retirement years are a time for nurturing hobbies, spending quality time with loved ones, and embracing a slower pace of Life.

6. **Rest for Medically Weak or Affected Organs**

    Chronic conditions affecting vital organs such as the kidneys, prostate, or liver require diligent care and sufficient rest. Overexertion can compromise organ function, worsen underlying health issues. Regular monitoring through medical check-ups, adhering to prescribed treatments, and avoiding behaviors and habits that strain these organs—such as excessive alcohol consumption or a high-protein diet—are critical. Rest does not only mean physical relaxation but also avoiding stressors that may worsen medical conditions.

Conclusion

In conclusion, aging gracefully requires a thoughtful and comprehensive approach to health, one that prioritizes balance and moderation in every aspect of life. For seniors, particularly those over 70, the importance of adhering to proper physiotherapy routines, maintaining a healthy and appropriate diet, protecting oneself from extreme weather conditions, avoiding overexertion, and giving vital organs the rest they need cannot be overlooked. By taking a proactive approach to these factors, seniors can enhance their quality of life, minimize health risks, and continue to enjoy their later years with vitality and fulfillment. These strategies, paired with regular medical guidance and self-care, can empower individuals to navigate their golden years with vitality and resilience.

Chapter 11

Suggestions and Conclusion

Aging is an inevitable and multifaceted journey, filled with both challenges and opportunities. This book has explored various dimensions of aging—ranging from physical and mental health to emotional well-being and spiritual growth. Through the personal stories of Alice, Walter, Lena, Rajiv and real life stories in chapter-9, we have come to understand that aging is shaped not only by genetics but also by environment, lifestyle choices, and mindset. These narratives emphasise the importance of a holistic approach to aging—one that nurtures resilience, fosters social connections, stimulates the mind, and nourishes the spirit.

Lessons from Personal Stories

- **Alice's Story** highlights the crucial role of family support in managing memory loss and demonstrates how a nurturing environment fosters emotional well-being.

- **Walter's Experience** reinforces the significance of maintaining meaningful social connections, which are vital for sustaining happiness and mental health as we age.

- **Lena's Journey** reveals that genetic predispositions are not a life sentence— with the right mindset and proactive care, individuals can overcome health challenges and live vibrant, fulfilling lives.

- **Rajiv's Focus on Community** underscores the importance of social bonds in both emotional and physical well-being, especially during later years.

- His life was a testament to the power of internal strength, and an example of determination and willpower. He was always adjusting to the needs of others and ensuring that he never became a burden.

- **The story of Dadaji** is not just one of personal triumph but a living example of how we should face life's challenges. His life, full of unwavering spiritualism, determination, and discipline, continues to be inspiration of hope and inspiration for our entire family. His legacy of strength, grace, and devotion to family and faith lives on in all of us.

- **The story of Mr. Vithal** offers invaluable lessons in resilience, strength, positive attitude and very strong will power – God helps those who help themselves, God helps those people who work on their problems and never blame their bad luck or blame others for their problems.

- **The Story of Dr. (Mrs.) Kiran Shingari** stands as a testament to the power of love, care, and support within a family, encouraging others to recognize the importance of these elements in fostering resilience and promoting overall well-being.

Key Suggestions & Recommendations for Seniors

Seniors can significantly enhance their quality of life by embracing a balance between nature and nurture. While genetics may influence certain aspects of aging, our environment and personal choices have a profound effect on overall well-being. Here are several strategies to help seniors maintain a fulfilling life around the age of 70:

1. **Surround Yourself with Positive Environments**

   Engage with supportive people and participate in activities that engage both mind and body. A positive, enriching environment boosts emotional and mental health.

2. **Engage in Lifelong Learning**

   Continuously seek out new skills, hobbies, and challenges to stimulate the brain. Lifelong learning not only enhances cognitive function but also promotes overall mental well-being.

3. **Prioritize Physical and Mental Health**

   Actively manage your health through balanced nutrition, physical activity, and regular health screenings. Preventive care and an active lifestyle can reduce the impact of age-related diseases like cardiovascular issues, strokes, and cancers. Mental health is equally important—regular emotional support and care can mitigate many age-related challenges.

4. **Cultivate Resilience and Adaptability**

Aging inevitably brings change. Embrace transitions with flexibility and resilience, whether adjusting to health issues or seeking help when needed. Developing adaptability is essential for maintaining mental and emotional balance in later years.

5. **Foster Spirituality and Mindfulness**

Spiritual practices such as meditation, prayer, or mindfulness techniques significantly contribute to mental and physical health. They reduce stress, enhance cognitive function, promote restful sleep, and stabilize emotions. Furthermore, spirituality fosters deeper connections within communities, reducing isolation and enhancing life satisfaction.

6. **Encourage Inter-generational Conversations**

Sharing wisdom with younger generations not only benefits them but also strengthens family bonds. For seniors, it offers a sense of purpose and fulfillment, enriching their later years and contributing to a greater sense of joy and meaning.

Conclusion

Aging is not a process to be feared, but one to be embraced—an opportunity for growth, fulfillment, and continued contribution to society. A healthy, happy life in later years depends on proactive steps such as staying physically active, nurturing mental well-being, cultivating spiritual peace, and fostering strong social connections. By adopting these strategies, seniors can enjoy a life that is not only longer but also richer in experiences, fulfillment, and resilience. With the right mindset, support systems, and lifestyle choices, older adults can continue to lead meaningful and purposeful lives. **Aging, when approached with awareness and intention, offers opportunities for deeper connection, growth, and joy, making each stage of life a meaningful journey.**

The Secrets of Old Age

To All Retired Friends...

People are not born great,

their thoughts make them great.

It is purity and simplicity of thoughts and actions,

that separate great person from the rest.

1. **SAFEGUARD YOUR FOUR PRICELESS ASSETS**

   A. Your old body - pay more attention to health, **you can only rely on yourself in this.**

   B. Retirement funds - **money that you have earned, it is best to keep them yourself.**

   C. Your old companion - treasure and replenish every moment with your better half, **one of you will leave first, WHO?**

D. Your old friends - seize every opportunities to meet up with your friends,

    such opportunities will become rare as time goes by.

2. **WORRY IS POINTLESS**

    A. If worries can cure your sickness, then go ahead and worry!

    B. If worries can prolong your life, then go ahead and worry!

    C. If worries can exchange for happiness, then go ahead and worry!

        If none of these outcomes are possible, why waste your time and energy on worry?

3. **ENJOY YOUR LIFE TO ITS FULLEST**

    A. Do not wait till you cannot even walk just to be sorry and to regret!

    B. As long as it is physically possible, visit places you wish to visit.

4. **AVAIL EVERY OPPORTUNITIY**

    Whenever you have the chance, meet with old classmates, colleagues, and friends. These gathering are not just about food - **they are about cherishing the moments you have left together.**

5. **SPEND YOUR MONEY WISELY - BUT DON'T HESITATE TO USE IT**

    A. Money in the bank may not always be there for you.

B. When the time comes, don't hesitate to spend on yourself-treat yourself well.

C. Eat what you love and enjoy it.

D. Focus on healthy foods, but don't be overly restricted.

E. Indulge in less healthy foods occasionally-enjoy life in moderation.

F. Most importantly, focus on your happiness.

6. ACCEPT DEATH AS A NATURAL PART OF LIFE

A. Face illness with optimism. Whether poor or rich, every human being goes through birth, aging, sickness and death are universal experiences. It is the cycle of life.

B. Do not fear sickness or death. Settle your affairs in advance, so you can leave this world without regrets.

C. Let the doctors handle your body, trust GOD or NATURE to oversee your life, but always take control of your own emotion/mood.

D. Ensure your will is in safe place.

7. THE TRUTH ABOUT LIFE

Life flows Forward like a river - it never moves backward. Make it meaningful. Smile often and laugh wholeheartedly, and spread happiness wherever you go.

Nothing is more refreshing,

than a healthful morning that,

calms your mind and gives you reasons
to smile and be happy.

—*Dr. M.K. Shingari*

This new year 2025 Message was shared with my friends and loved ones. I feel it is a message worth including in my book for seniors aged 70 and above.

To promote healthy aging I also recommend embracing the following habits.

- Keep your brain active.

- Prevent falls

- Exercises regularly & eat a healthy diets

- Get sufficient rest

- Find purpose in life

- Stay active and engaged with life

—*Dr. M.K. Shingari*

Appendix 2

Dangerous Age Group

The Criticality of the Age Between 70 and 79

The age group between 70 and 79 is often considered a pivotal period, it is very important because other things depend on it. This period in the human lifespan is very critical and known as **"Dangerous Age Group"**. In countries like Israel and Japan, where longevity is very high and studied, according to them this decade (70-79) is recognized as a particularly **critical and troublesome time.** Many individuals face heightened health risks, psychological challenges, and social transitions during these years.

After entering the age of 80, diseases like hypertension, diabetes, hyperlipidemia (hardening of the arteries) etc. will decline, and the mental and physical help may return to the level of 60-69 years life span. Many individuals face high health risks, psychological challenges, and social transitions during these years. Understanding the factors that make this age group significant can help them navigate from this period effectively.

Physiological Challenges

Aging naturally brings about a decline in bodily functions, and this decline often becomes more pronounced in the 70s. Chronic conditions such as cardiovascular diseases, diabetes, arthritis, and respiratory illnesses are common during this period. **The immune system weakens,** making individuals more susceptible to infections and slower to recover from illnesses.

Cognitive decline is another critical concern. While not everyone develops dementia or Alzheimer's disease, the risk of such neurodegenerative conditions increases significantly. Even without severe cognitive impairments, many individuals experience memory lapses and slower processing speeds, which can impact daily life.

Furthermore, the body's ability to repair itself diminishes. Fractures from falls, for instance, can lead to prolonged recovery periods or complications, further threatening independence and quality of life. These physical vulnerabilities underscore why the 70s are considered a dangerous decade for many.

Psychological and Emotional Struggles

The psychological toll of aging often intensifies during the 70s. This period is marked by significant life transitions, including retirement, the loss of loved ones, and changes in social roles. These shifts can lead to feelings of isolation, depression, and anxiety.

A sense of purpose is crucial for mental well-being, but many people in their 70s struggle to redefine their roles in a society that often undervalues the elderly. The loss of professional identity and reduced physical capabilities can lead to feelings of that I am not having qualities and abilities necessary to do something and cope with life further and loses self-confidence.

Social Dynamics and Support Systems

Social connections play a crucial role in the well-being of individuals in their 70s. However, this age group often experiences a shrinking social circle due to the deaths of friends and family members, physical limitations, or mobility issues. Isolation can aggravate / worsen. both physical and mental health problems, creating a vicious cycle.

Cultural attitudes toward aging can also influence the experience of this decade. In countries like Japan, where respect for elders is deeply ingrained, social structures and traditions provide some support. In contrast, societies that prioritize youth may inadvertently marginalize older individuals, leaving them feeling disconnected and undervalued.

Coping Strategies and Interventions

To cope up these crucial 10-year health care from 70 to 79 years is to follow some simple steps called as **"Doing ten ones every day"** and this will help to navigate more smoothly through the **"Dangerous Age Group"** stage of your life.

1. **Five litre container of water**

    Water is "the best and cheapest health drink".

    You must drink a glass of water during the following three times/occasions each day:

First Glass:

    After getting out of bed, you can drink a glass of water on an empty stomach. Lukewarm water will be more beneficial.

    Because of our invisible sweating and urine secretion during sleep, we lose a lot of water. Even if we don't feel thirsty after getting up, the body liquids will still be thick due to lack of water. Therefore, after getting out of bed, you must drink water as soon as possible.

Second Glass:

    A glass of water after exercise

    The right amount of exercise is one of the cornerstones of longevity, especially for the elderly, and **more attention should be paid to effective and reasonable exercise.** However, after exercise, special attention should be paid to replenishing water. During exercise, sweat takes away electrolytes and consumes more energy. If you don't pay attention, it is prone to hypoglycemia after exercise, and even cause syncope (a loss of consciousness for a short period of time). **Therefore, after the exercise, it is recommended that the old people drink water to which a small pinch of salt and sugar can be added and dissolved if you wish.**

Third Glass:

A glass of water before going to bed / sleeping.

When people are asleep, sweat glands are still draining water. When the body's water is reduced too much, the blood viscosity is increased. A glass of water before going to bed can effectively reduce the blood viscosity and may even slow down the appearance of aging. Helps against Angina, myocardial infarction and other diseases.

2. **A bowl of *Dalia* / Oats cooked in milk (Porridge)**

China Daily Online published a 14-year study conducted by Harvard University on 100,000 people. It found that a bowl of about 28 grams of whole grain cereal porridge per day can reduce mortality by 9% and reduce the chance of getting cardiovascular diseases.

Each volunteer was in good physical condition when he participated in the study in 1984, but in the 2010 feedback survey, more than 26,000 volunteers had passed away.

It was found that those volunteers who regularly ate whole grains such as porridge, brown rice, corn and buckwheat seem to have avoided most diseases, especially heart diseases.

3. A cup of milk

Milk is known as "White blood" and it is so to the human body. Its nutritional value is well known with a lot of calcium, fat and protein.

The recommended daily intake of milk and dairy products is 300 grams.

4. An egg

Eggs can be said to be the most suitable food for human consumption. The body's absorption rate of egg protein can be as high as 98%.!!

5. An apple

Modern research believes that apples have the effects of lowering cholesterol, losing weight, preventing cancer, preventing aging, enhancing memory, and making the skin smooth and soft.

The health benefits of different colored apples are different:

Red apples have the effect of lowering blood lipids and softening blood vessels

Green apple has the effect of nourishing liver and detoxifying, and can fight depression, so it is more suitable for young people to eat.

Yellow apples have a good effect on protecting vision.

6. **An onion**

The Onion has a very high nutritional value and has many functions, including helping to lower blood sugar, lowering cholesterol, preventing cancer, protecting cardiovascular and cerebrovascular diseases, and also anti- bacteria, preventing colds, and supplementing calcium and bones. Eat onions at least three or four times a week.

7. **A piece of fish**

Chinese Nutritionists have warned that eating "Four legs" is worse than eating "two legs", eating "Two legs" is worse than eating "No legs."

"Four legs" mainly refers to pigs, cattle, and mutton. Eating too much of these meats is not conducive to weight loss and lowering blood fat;

"Two legs" mainly refers to poultry such as chicken, duck, goose, etc., which are good meat foods;

"No legs" mainly refers to fish and various vegetables. The protein contained in fish is easily digested and absorbed. The amount of unsaturated fatty acids in the fat, especially polyunsaturated fatty acids, is relatively good for the body.

8. **Gentle walking**

This has a magical anti-aging effect. When adults walk (about 1 kilometre or less) regularly for more than 12 weeks, they will achieve the effect of correct posture and waist circumference, and the body becomes strong and not easily tired.

In addition, walking exercise is also beneficial to treat headache, back pain, shoulder pain, etc., and can promote sleep.

Experts believe that a 30-minute walk a day can get rid of the danger of "Adult disease". People who take 10,000 steps a day will have a lower chance of developing cardiovascular and cerebrovascular disease.

9. **A hobby**

Having a hobby, whether it is raising flowers, raising birds, collecting stamps, fishing, or painting, singing, playing chess, and traveling, can help the elderly to maintain extensive contact with society and nature. This broadens the horizons of interest of the elderly. They will love and cherish life.

10. **Good Mood**

Old people should maintain **positive emotions** as these are extremely important to their good health. Common chronic diseases which affect the elderly are closely related to the **negative emotions** of the elderly:

Many patients with coronary heart disease have angina and myocardial infarction due to stimulation of adverse emotions, resulting in sudden death;

"Bad temper" leads to high blood pressure. In prolonged and severe cases, this can cause stroke, heart failure, sudden death, etc.;

Negative Emotions such as anger, anxiety, and grief can cause blood sugar levels to rise, causing metabolic disorders in the body.

This shows how important it is to have a good mood!

Conclusion

The decade between 70 and 79 is undeniably a critical phase of life, marked by significant challenges. By addressing the physical, emotional, and social aspects of aging, individuals can transform this potentially dangerous period of life into safe period like **before 70-79**, and enjoy the rest of the remaining life. Awareness, preparation, and support are key to navigate these crucial years with dignity and grace.

Appendix 3

Yoga Exercises for Seniors

As we age, maintaining physical health and mental well-being becomes increasingly important, and the practice of yoga has emerged as a highly beneficial tool for senior citizens, particularly those over the age of 70. Regular physical activity, such as yoga, can significantly enhance the quality of life for older adults by improving flexibility, strength, balance, and mental clarity, all of which tend to decline with age. I will explore the benefits of yoga for senior citizens above 70 and provide recommendations for specific yoga exercises that cater to their needs.

Benefits of Yoga for Senior Citizens

* **Improved Flexibility and Joint Mobility:**   One of the primary benefits of yoga for seniors is the improvement in flexibility. Aging often results in stiffness and reduced range of motion in joints and muscles. Yoga involves gentle stretching, which can help maintain or even restore flexibility, thereby reducing the risk of

injury and promoting better mobility. Regular practice of yoga helps seniors maintain and regain flexibility in key areas like the spine, hips, and shoulders, elbow, wrist joint and knee etc. etc. enabling them to perform everyday tasks more easily.

- **Enhanced Balance and Coordination:** Falls are a significant concern for seniors, and balance issues become more common with age. <u>Yoga focuses on postures that engage the core muscles, improve coordination, and strengthen the lower body.</u> Through consistent practice, seniors can enhance their ability to maintain balance, which helps in preventing falls and the injuries that often result from them.

- **Increased Strength and Endurance:** Yoga can help older adults build strength, particularly in areas that may have weakened over time, such as legs, arms and the back. By holding postures for longer duration and engaging in controlled movements, seniors can develop muscle tone and endurance. This can lead to better posture, improved stamina, and greater overall physical functioning.

- **Mental Well-Being and Stress Relief:** Yoga incorporates breathing exercises (*Pranayama*) and meditation, which can have a profound impact on mental health. For seniors, <u>these techniques are especially valuable in reducing stress, anxiety, and depression.</u> The meditative aspects of yoga help calm the mind, improve focus, and encourage mindfulness.

Additionally, regular yoga practice can promote better sleep and enhance cognitive function, which is particularly important for seniors as they age.

* **Improved Circulation and Cardiovascular Health:** The physical postures in yoga help stimulate circulation and can improve Cardiovascular health. Many yoga poses increase blood flow to vital organs and muscles, helping to maintain a healthy heart and lower blood pressure.

For seniors with conditions such as hypertension or arthritis, yoga offers a low-impact form of exercise that improves overall circulation and heart health without putting undue strain on the body.

Recommended Yoga Exercises

While yoga is beneficial for people of all ages, seniors should focus on exercises that are gentle on the body, improve flexibility, strength, and balance, and promote relaxation. Below are a few recommended yoga poses/ exercises. These exercises can be done either on a chair or on a yoga mat, depending on the individual's mobility and comfort level.

All exercises shall be initially practice under the guidance of a trained teacher before practicing these on your own.

Never overexert yourself during any exercises as every individual is unique and has different limitations.

Always take rest in between two exercises. Exercises in sitting postures:

A. Hand Exercises

1. Stretch hands straight and

   a. open and close the palms 10-20 times

   b. Rotate wrists clockwise and anti-clockwise 10-20 times each

   c. Bend hands upwards from elbows 10-20 times.

   d. Raise hands above your head 10 times

2. Put Hands on the knees and rotate shoulders 10 times first in clockwise and then in anti-clockwise direction.

3. Stretch hands on your sides and clap for 40-50 times

B. Leg Exercises

1. Stretch Legs while sitting on the chair and

   a. Raise fingers of feet up and down 15-20 times

   b. Bend feet up and down for 15-20 times

   c. Rotate feet clockwise and anti-clockwise 10 times each

2. In sitting posture itself, move both legs like march past for 40- 50 times

C. Neck Exercises

Sit straight on the chair and

a. Bend your neck on left and right side slowly for 8-10 times

b. Bend your neck up and down 8-10 times

c. Keeping eyes closed, rotate your neck alternately clockwise and anti-clockwise very slowly for 4-5 times each.

D. Eyes Exercises

Sit straight on the chair and stretch your one hand and raise one finger in front of your eyes. Focus both the eyes on the finger.

a. Slowly shift finger left and right while moving your eye balls simultaneously focusing eye balls on the finger 8-10 times.

   DO NOT MOVE YOUR NECK DURING THESE EYE EXERCISES

b. Move the finger up and down simultaneously moving your eye balls focusing on the finger 8-10 times

c. Move the finger in circular clockwise motion and anti-clockwise motion alternatively 4-5 times each while rotating eye balls along with the rotating finger.

E. Chanting 'OM'

Take deep breath and exhale it slowly by chanting 'OM'. Repeat this three times after taking a rest of 1 minute in between.

- **Tad Asana (Mountain Pose)** improves blood circulation throughout the body, which can help to reduce swelling and improve overall health, it reduces stress and anxiety: This pose helps to calm the mind and reduce stress and anxiety, making it an excellent pose for relaxation and stress relief. It involves standing tall with feet 3-4 inches apart, arms at the sides, and the body weight evenly distributed. The focus is on grounding the feet and lengthening the spine. For seniors, this pose can be done while holding onto a chair or a wall for support. This simple pose enhances alignment and promotes mindfulness (Concentrate and do deep breathing).

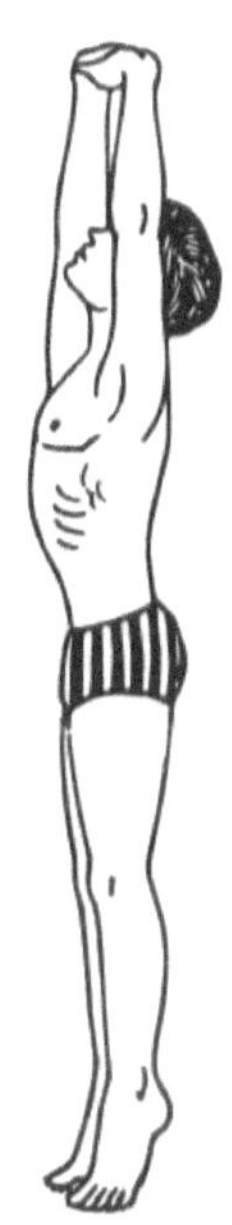

  Benefits: Improves posture, balance, and awareness of the body.

- *Utkat Asana (Chair Pose)* is considered to be one of the best *asana*. It strengthens the toes, the joints and the muscles of the feet. This technique is explained below.

  Technique: Stand with the legs together. Raise the body on the heels and bring the arms straight over the

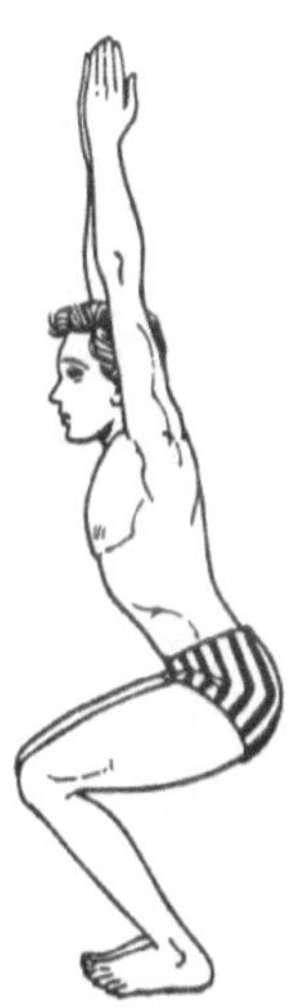

head and join the palms. Then slowly lower the trunk. This *asana* does not require much strength to practice it. For seniors, this can be modified by sitting in a sturdy chair and lifting the arms overhead.

Benefits: Strengthens the muscles of the wrists, the feet and legs. It also improves balance, and tones the body.

- ***Marjary Asana* (Cat-Cow Stretch)** Inhale deeply while curving your lower back and bringing your head up, tilting your pelvis up like a "cow." Exhale deeply and bring your 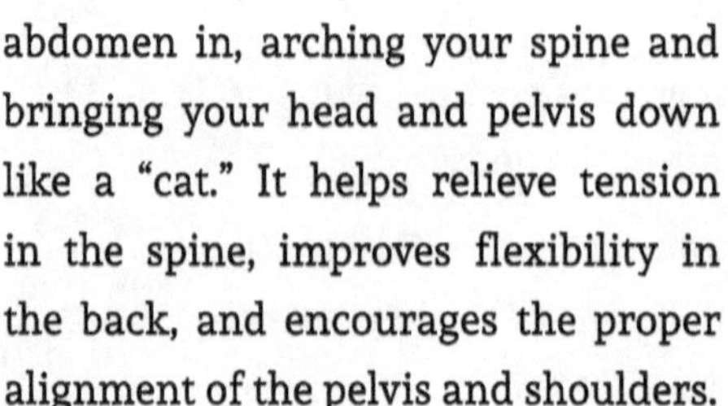 abdomen in, arching your spine and bringing your head and pelvis down like a "cat." It helps relieve tension in the spine, improves flexibility in the back, and encourages the proper alignment of the pelvis and shoulders.

Benefits: Improves spinal flexibility, eases back pain, and promotes better posture.

* **Vruksh Asana (Tree Pose)** This Pose is an excellent balance pose that helps strengthen the legs, improve focus, and increase stability. The individual stands on one leg, placing the sole of the other foot against the inner thigh or calf (avoiding the knee), while bringing the hands together and extending them overhead. If difficulty is experienced to balance the body on one leg, take the support of a wall. **Seniors with body balancing problem shall NEVER attempt it as one may fall during this exercise.**

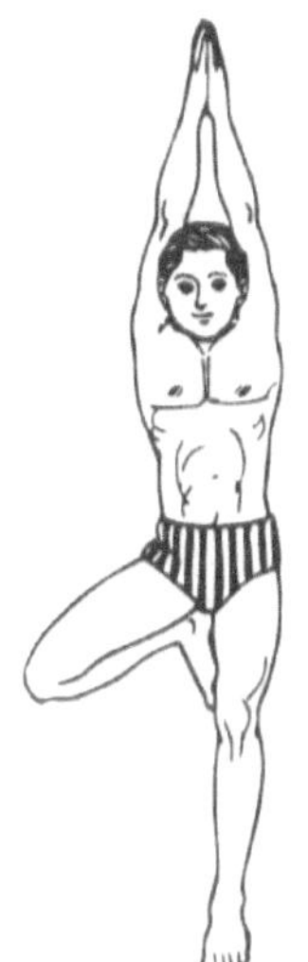

  Benefits: This tones up all the joints of the body. It supplies blood to the blood vessels of the toes, the knee, the elbows in sufficient quantity and improves concentration.

* **Paschimottan Asana (Seated Forward Fold)** This pose stretches the back, hamstrings, and calves. Seniors can practice this stretch 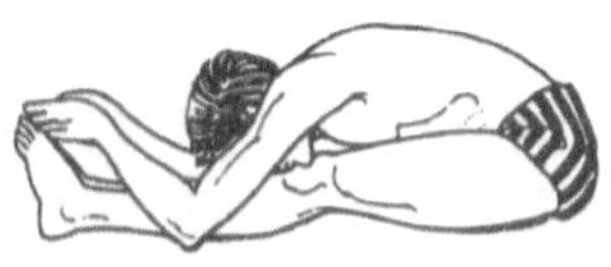 seated in a chair, hinging forward from the hips to reach towards the

feet. The key is to avoid straining and to focus on gentle stretching.

Benefits: Stretches the back and hamstrings, promotes relaxation, and improves flexibility.

- ***Setubandh Asana* (Bridge Pose)** Seniors can perform this exercise by lying on their back with feet flat on the floor and knees bent. By lifting the hips towards the ceiling and 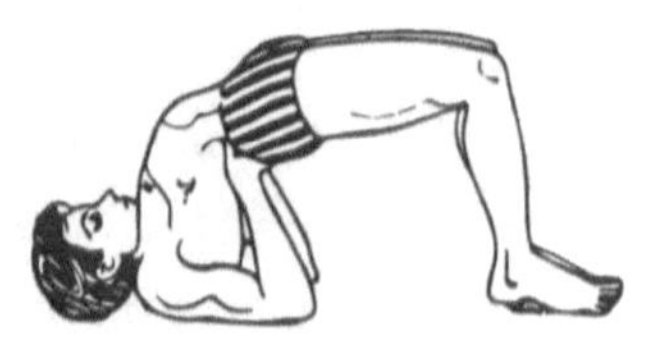 squeezing the glutes, seniors can strengthen their lower body and improve posture.

  Benefits: Strengthens the large muscles of buttocks and back, the neck, elbows and hands. Also opens the chest, expel excess gases and cures indigestion. This asana makes the spine flexible and active.

- ***Shavasana:*** *Shavasana* is a resting pose commonly used in between asanas as well as at the end of a yoga session. It involves lying flat on the back with arms and legs extended and the body fully relaxed. One shall inhale and exhale very slowly while focusing mind on feeling happy and healthy. This pose allows seniors to rest and absorb the benefits of their practice, reducing stress and promoting mental clarity.

Benefits: Relieves tension, promotes relaxation, and helps in mental rejuvenation.

Conclusion

Yoga is a powerful tool for promoting physical and mental well-being for every age group specially for seniors above 70. By incorporating simple, low-impact exercises into their daily routine, seniors can improve flexibility, balance, strength, and overall health. Yoga also offers significant mental health benefits, including stress relief and enhanced cognitive function. With the right modifications and guidance, yoga can be safely practiced by seniors, helping them lead healthier, more active lives as they age.

MEDITATION FOR SENIORS

As people age, maintaining mental and emotional well-being becomes just as important as physical health. For seniors above the age of 70, meditation has emerged as a powerful tool for improving quality of life and many more benefits as under:

- Improves memory, mental clarity, and overall cognitive function.

- Reduces stress, anxiety, and depression, leading to better emotional well-being.

- Promotes deeper, more restful sleep and improves overall sleep patterns.

- Helps regulate emotions, improve mood, and enhance emotional resilience.

- Increases self-awareness, acceptance, and a sense of peace with aging.

Explanation of Benefits of Meditation

Improved Cognitive Function and Memory: As seniors age, cognitive decline, such as memory loss and slower processing speed, can become common challenges. Meditation has been shown to help improve focus, memory, and cognitive function. By regularly practicing mindfulness and attention-based techniques, seniors can stimulate brain activity and reduce age-related memory issues. Studies have shown that meditation can enhance the size of certain **Brain Regions** involved in memory and cognitive control, such as the **Hippocampus** (a part of your brain responsible for your memory and learning.) and **Prefrontal Cortex** (a part of your brain responsible for executive functions, such as planning, decision making, working memory, personality expression, moderating social behavior and controlling certain aspects of speech and language.)

- **Reduced Stress and Anxiety:** Seniors often face stress related to aging, health problems, or loss of loved ones. Chronic stress can negatively impact physical and mental health, leading to issues like insomnia, high blood pressure, and depression. Meditation has been proven to reduce stress by promoting relaxation and activating the body's parasympathetic nervous system, which is responsible for the "rest and digest" response. Mindfulness meditation, in particular, teaches individuals to focus on the present moment and detach from worries, helping to alleviate anxiety and emotional distress.

- **Improved Sleep Quality:** Sleep problems, such as insomnia or disrupted sleep cycles, are common in older adults. Meditation helps calm the mind and relax the body, making it easier to fall asleep and stay asleep. By incorporating meditation into their evening routine, seniors can reduce the mental chatter that often interferes with sleep. Guided relaxation techniques and deep-breathing exercises can help promote restful sleep and improve overall sleep quality.

Keep your mind in complete rest mode 2-3 hours before your bed time. This can be done by switching off your TV, Mobile etc. though a soft music at low volume can be put on.

- **Enhanced Emotional Regulation**: Aging can sometimes lead to emotional challenges, including feelings of loneliness, sadness, or frustration. Meditation helps seniors cultivate mindfulness, which in turn fosters emotional regulation. Practicing self-awareness through meditation enables seniors to identify their emotions without judgment, allowing them to respond more calmly and thoughtfully to challenging situations. This heightened emotional intelligence can enhance their relationships with others and improve their overall emotional resilience.

- **Increased Self-Awareness and Acceptance**: Meditation encourages introspection and self-reflection, which can lead to greater self-awareness. As seniors age, they may struggle with feelings of loss or the changing nature of their lives. Meditation helps individuals process these changes by promoting a sense of acceptance and understanding of the present moment. Seniors who practice meditation are better able to cultivate a sense of peace with their past and present, leading to greater life satisfaction and emotional contentment.

- **Reduced Risk of Age-Related Illnesses**: Chronic illnesses such as hypertension, heart disease, and diabetes are more prevalent among the elderly. Meditation has been shown to have positive effects on physical health, including lowering blood pressure, improving heart rate variability, and reducing inflammation in the body. By reducing stress and promoting relaxation, meditation may also help to reduce the risk of stress-related illnesses that are more common in senior citizens.

Recommended Meditation Practices

While meditation offers numerous benefits, it is essential for seniors to engage in practices that are gentle, accessible, and suited to their individual needs. Below are some meditation techniques that can be especially helpful for seniors over 70, each designed to promote relaxation, mental clarity, and overall well-being.

A. **Mindfulness Meditation:** It is a simple yet effective practice that involves focusing attention on the present moment, observing thoughts and sensations without judgment. Seniors can practice mindfulness by paying attention to their breath, bodily sensations, or the sounds around them. The goal is to become aware of thoughts and emotions as they arise, without getting caught up in them. This practice can be done sitting comfortably, either in a chair or on a cushion.

How to Practice: Sit in a comfortable position, close the eyes, and bring attention to your breath.

Inhale and exhale slowly, noticing the sensations in the body with each breath. When the mind wanders, gently guide your focus back to the breath without judgment.

Benefits: Increases awareness, reduces stress, and enhances cognitive function.

B. **Guided Meditation:** For seniors who find it difficult to meditate on their own, guided meditation is an excellent option. In guided meditation, an instructor or audio recording leads the participant through a series of instructions, often focusing on relaxation, visualization, or mindfulness. This type of meditation can be particularly helpful for seniors who need additional support to stay focused during their practice.

How to Practice: Find a comfortable and quiet space. Listen to a guided meditation recording that leads you through relaxation techniques or visualization exercises. These can be found as 'Online Applications' specifically designed for seniors.

Benefits: Helps with focus, and promotes relaxation.

C. **Breathing Exercises (*Pranayama*):** These are simple practices that focus on controlled breathing to calm the mind and body. Seniors can practice deep breathing or alternate nostril breathing to reduce stress, increase oxygen flow, and promote relaxation. These exercises are easy to perform and can be done seated or lying down position.

How to Practice: Try deep belly breathing by inhaling deeply through the nose, holding the breath for a few seconds, and then exhaling slowly through the mouth. Alternatively, try alternate nostril breathing, where one nostril is closed while breathing through the other.

Benefits: Reduces stress, improves lung function, and promotes relaxation.

D. **Body Scan Meditation:** It is a technique that involves systematically focusing on different parts of the body, noticing any tension or discomfort. This practice helps seniors become more aware of their bodies, relax tense muscles, and promote a sense of physical relaxation. The body scan can be practiced lying down or seated.

How to Practice: Lie down in a comfortable position, close your eyes, and bring attention to each part of the body, starting from the toes and moving upwards. Notice any sensations, tension, or areas of discomfort, and breathe into those areas to release tension.

Benefits: Increases body awareness, reduces tension, and promotes relaxation.

Conclusion

Meditation can be an invaluable practice for senior citizens, particularly those over the age of 70. By incorporating meditation into their daily routine, seniors can enjoy a range of physical and mental health benefits, including reduced stress, improved cognitive function, better emotional regulation, and enhanced sleep quality. The simplicity and accessibility of meditation make it an ideal practice for older adults, and the various techniques—such as mindfulness, guided meditation, and breathing exercises—offer options to suit individual needs. Through regular meditation practice, seniors can cultivate a sense of peace, mindfulness, and overall well-being, enriching their lives as they age.

SUPER BRAIN YOGA (SBY)

Super Brain Yoga is a transformative technique that integrates physical movement, mindfulness, and energy healing to optimise brain function and overall well-being. With consistent practice, you can unlock the full potential of your mind and lead a more balanced, fulfilling life.

The meditative aspect of Super Brain Yoga promotes emotional balance and reduces stress. With regular practice, you may experience a sense of calmness and clarity, enhancing your overall quality of life.

In Tamil Nadu, Super Brain Yoga is referred to as *Thorpi Karnam or Thoppukarnam*. The technique combines acupressure, breath-work, and physical exercises like squatting. It is reported that SBY strengthens the immune system and, in turn, enhances cognitive function.This ancient healing technique was popularized in the Western world by Grand Master Choa Kok Sui.

Recently, I came across two articles on Super Brain Yoga published in the European Journal of Cardiovascular Medicine. The first, titled 'Study of Effect on Attention Span of Adolescent Males', was authored by Associate Professors Shilpa and Sunita from the Department of Physiology, JJM Medical College, Davangere, Karnataka, and published on May 30, 2024.

The second article, 'The Effect of Super Brain Yoga' on the Cognitive Function of Hemodialysis Patients, was authored by Mahdi Babakhani, Kobra Rahzani, Davood

Hekmatpou, and Vida Sheykh, and published in September 2024.

Super Brain Yoga, as the name implies, keeps your mind busy and sharp, allowing you to get the most out of it. This yoga technique is a form of brain training and exercise that increases mindfulness, focus, and supports cognitive function. Isn't it true that with an active and sharp mind, one can resolve almost all of life's challenges?

Introduction

The human brain is a powerful and complex organ with countless neuronal connections. It is even more sophisticated than any existing computer. There are around 86 billion neurons in the human brain.

Many yogic practices are studied and practiced to improve brain capacity; one of these is **Super Brain Yoga**. It is a very simple yet effective technique to energise and recharge brain cells. This practice is based on the theory of subtle energy (*prana*) and ear acupuncture. It was first popularized by Master Choa Kok Sui as a method to recharge and energize the brain.

Super Brain Yoga involves holding the earlobes with the fingers, crossing the arms over the chest, and performing 14 squats with coordinated breathing. SBY is a simple yet effective method that benefits not only students but also adults seeking holistic well-being. This exercise cleanses and energises energy centers called *chakras*, which are vital for efficient brain function. When energy from the lower *chakras* moves upward, it transforms into *pranic* energy associated with spirituality. Since the upper *chakras* control and energise the brain, *pranic* energy is used to enhance brain function.

Mindfulness and Meditation in Super Brain Yoga

When combined with mindfulness and meditation, Super Brain Yoga can significantly boost cognition and emotional well-being. Cognition is the mental process of thinking, learning, remembering, being aware of surroundings, and using judgment.

Here are steps to guide your practice:

+ **Focus on the Present Moment (Selective Attention):** Selective attention is a cognitive process that involves focusing on a particular object or stimulus for a period of time while simultaneously ignoring distractions and irrelevant information. This ability allows us to tune out insignificant details and concentrate on what is important. Individuals with short attention spans may struggle to focus on tasks without being easily distracted. During each posture and breathing exercise, concentrate fully on your present.

+ **Observe Sensations Without Judgment:** Notice the sensations in your body, the rhythm of your breath, and the flow of thoughts in your mind.

- **Connect with Your Inner Self:** Reduce distractions and foster a state of tranquility (Calmness) through deep introspection.

- **Optimize Brain Stimulation:** Pay close attention to precise movements for maximum cognitive benefits.

Benefits of Super Brain Yoga

Super Brain Yoga is a straightforward squatting exercise that does not involve twisting or turning the body. It promotes mental health, facilitates mental fitness, and supports brain development. Here are some of its benefits:

- **Improves Mental Agility and Creativity:** SBY enhances mental sharpness and fosters creative thinking.

- **Boosts Blood Circulation in the Brain:** This may result in improved memory and cognitive function.

- **Promotes Psychological Health:** SBY supports emotional well-being and reduces stress.

- **Helps with Neurological Conditions:** It benefits individuals with Dyslexia (Dyslexia is a learning disability that disrupts how your brain processes written language. People with dyslexia have trouble with reading and related skills.), ADHD (Attention Deficit Hyperactivity Disorder is a condition that affects people's behaviour. People with ADHD can seem restless, may have trouble concentrating and may act on impulse.), Dementia, and other neurological disorders.

- **Enhances Memory in Older Adults:** The practice significantly improves memory for daily tasks, such as finding keys.

- **Increases Calmness and Inner Peace:** SBY promotes mental clarity and helps balance emotions for a more stable and positive outlook.

- **Supports Holistic Health:** The technique aids in controlling appetite and maintaining overall well-being.

Dr. Joie P. Jones of the University of California researched the authenticity of Super Brain Yoga. His study demonstrated that the practice effectively activates acupuncture points on the ears, stimulating cognitive function.

Suggestions

Encourage older adults to participate in physical activities tailored to their abilities, such as walking, or strength training.

Foster strong social networks through community programs, social clubs, and family connections to reduce isolation.

Promote mindfulness and stress-reduction practices to help manage anxiety and depression.

Recommend cognitive exercises and lifelong learning to support brain health and maintain cognitive function.

Advocate for accessible mental health services that cater to the needs of older adults, including counselling, therapy, and support groups.

How to Do Superbrain Yoga

Super brain Yoga is a simple beneficial exercise that does not involve any complicated body twists or turns. It is designed to help improve aspects of your mental health such as concentration. Super brain yoga is a simple activity that involves touching the ears and doing squats.

Super Brain Yoga is a simple exercise said to enhance brain function by synchronizing the brain's hemispheres, improving focus, and boosting energy. It combines physical movement with breathing techniques and stimulation of acupressure points. Here's a detailed procedure along with descriptions for illustrations:

Steps to Perform Super Brain Yoga

1. Face East (Optional)

*   Stand facing East, especially during the morning, as it is believed to maximize energy alignment.

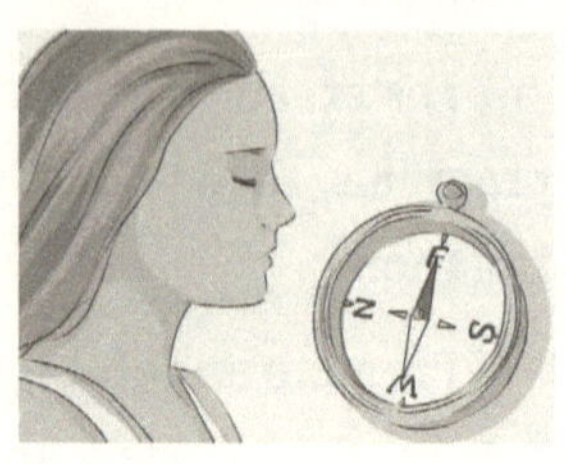

*   However, if you are elderly, you can face the North.

2. **Remove Jewelry**

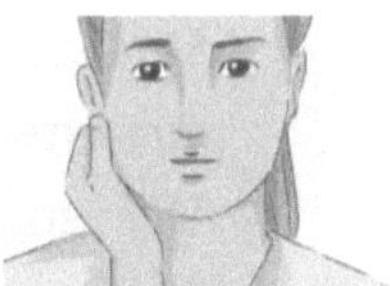

- Take off any jewelry or metallic items that may interfere with energy flow.

3. **Place Tongue on the Roof of Your Mouth**

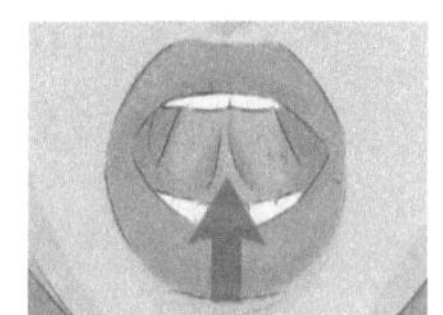

- Touch your tongue to the roof of your mouth and keep it there throughout the exercise. This is believed to complete an energy circuWit in your body.

- To start your routine, position your tongue correctly. During SBY, your tongue should be just behind your teeth on the roof of your mouth. It's the same place your tongue would be if you were about to say "La." Keep your tongue there for the whole exercise.

4. **Cross Arms Over Your Chest**

- Cross your arms in front of your chest, right hand touching your left earlobe and left hand touching your right earlobe.

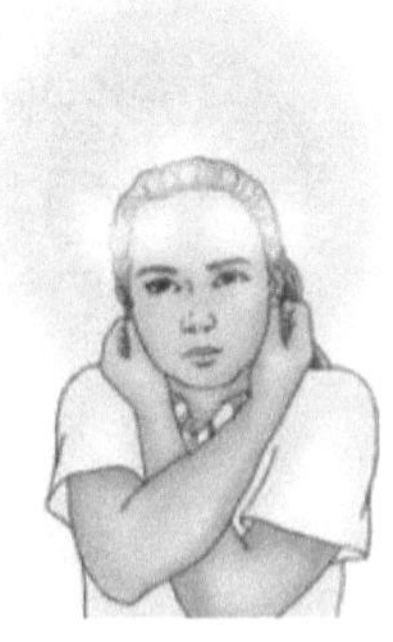

- Ensure your thumb is pressing on the front of the earlobe while your other fingers support the back.

5. Press and Hold the Earlobes

    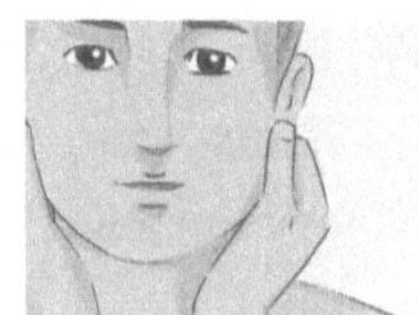

    - Apply gentle but firm pressure on both earlobes. This stimulates acupressure points connected to the brain.

6. Breathe Deeply

    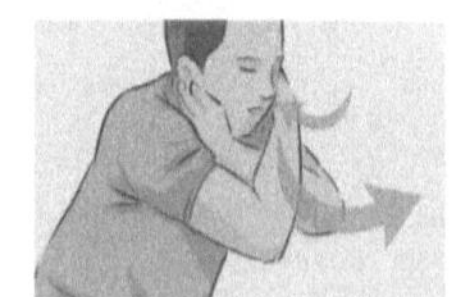

    - Inhale deeply through your nose as you squat down.

7. Perform Squats

    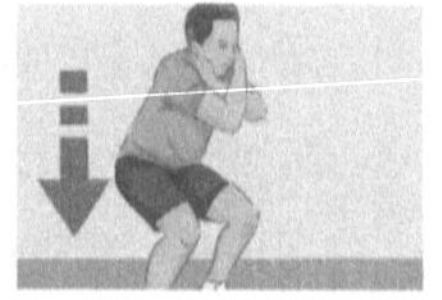

    - Exhale as you rise back to a standing position.

    - Repeat this squat movement 15–20 times.

    - Maintain the crossed-arm position and proper breathing rhythm throughout.

8. Release and Relax

    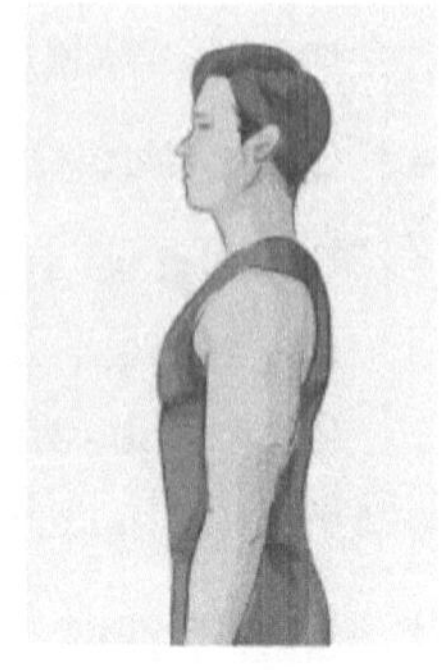

    - Once you've completed the squats, release your earlobes and let your arms relax by your sides.

    - Take a few deep breaths and observe how you feel.

Conclusion

Super Brain Yoga is a powerful tool for promoting physical and mental well-being for every age group specially for seniors above 70. It promotes mental health, facilitates mental fitness, and supports brain development. It also Improves Mental capability & Creativity, Psychological Health, Neurological Conditions and Boosts Blood Circulation in the Brain.

DO's and DO NOT's for Seniors Aged 70 and Above

1. In the House

(Especially to avoid Tripping and can make Seniors immobile)

DO's

- **Prevent Falls:** Prioritize fall prevention; injuries, especially to bones and muscles, can be challenging to recover from.

- **Employ Grip Mats:** Use non-slip shower mats while bathing to prevent slips and falls.

- **Use Western Toilets:** Western-style toilets with side railings make it easier

- **Install Railings:** Ensure railings are installed to assist with walking, particularly in areas such as bathrooms (near toilets and showers).

* **Use Firm Seating:** Opt for a straight-backed, firm chair for sitting to provide proper support.

* **Declutter the Bedroom:** Maintain a clean and clutter-free bedroom to allow safe movement and minimize the risk of tripping.

* **Adjust TV Placement:** Position your TV at an optimal distance to reduce eye strain and improve viewing comfort.

* **Sleep on a Firm Mattress:** A firm mattress provides better support for the back and reduces the risk of back pain.

* **Avoid Low Seating:** Do not use chairs or sofas that are too low, as they make it difficult to sit down and get up.

DO NOT's

* **Keep Bathroom Floors Wet:** Always Dry Bathroom Floors to prevent slipping.

* **Sleep Far from the Bathroom:** Position your bed close to the bathroom to minimize night time walking distance.

* **Install Dim Lighting:** Use Bright, clear lighting to enhance visibility and reduce fall risks.

* **Lift Heavy Items:** Avoid lifting or moving heavy objects to prevent strain or injury.

2. Outside the House

DO's:

* **Be Alert:** Watch your step and stay aware of your surroundings while walking and especially stepping on the stairs.

* **Wear Proper Shoes:** Use comfortable, firm shoes with good grip to avoid slipping.

* **Opt for Slopes:** Choose sloping paths instead of stairs whenever possible.

* **Plan Ahead:** Plan your outings and routes to reduce stress and ensure smooth navigation.

* **Carry Essentials:** Always have essential medications, water, and snacks with you. Diabetic patients must always carry sugar candy while going out.

* **Avoid Assisting Elders:** Do not take on the responsibility of helping other elderly individuals if it might strain you.

DO NOT's

* **Over commit:** Avoid engaging in too many activities at once.

* **Exhaust Yourself:** Do not exhaust yourself by overdoing physical or social activities.

* **Refrain Driving:** Refrain from driving if your vision is blurry or reaction times are slower.

- **Skip Planning:** Avoid spontaneous, unplanned activities or long-distance travel that might overexert you.

- **Avoid Assisting Others:** Do not take on the responsibility of helping other elderly individuals, it might strain you.

3. Eating

DO's

- **Eat Regularly:** Have smaller, easy to digest more frequent meals incorporating all food groups for proper nutrition and to maintain energy levels.

- **Consult a Nutritionist:** Seek professional advice for a meal plan tailored to your health needs.

- **Track Food Sensitivities:** Maintain a list of foods that upset your stomach and avoid them.

DO NOT TAKE

- **Rich Foods:** Steer clear of overly rich, fatty, or greasy foods.

- **Bloating Foods:** Avoid foods that cause gas or bloating, such as certain such as carbonated drinks.

- **Late-Night Meals:** Avoid eating too close to bedtime to support good digestion and sleep.

4. Socializing

DO's

♦ **Stay Connected:** Maintain regular contact with Friends and Family to reduce LONELINESS/ ISOLATION.

♦ **Foster Positive Relationships:** Surround yourself with people who bring joy and positivity.

♦ **Engage in Activities:** Join clubs or participate in hobbies and Social groups. Make an effort to attend social functions and community gatherings.

♦ **Be Friendly:** Cultivate a welcoming and good and courteous behaviour, which includes the way you stand, the way you talk, your facial expressions. Also give a friendly smile and look in the eyes while talking to them.

♦ **Attend Events:** Make an effort to attend social functions and community gatherings.

5. Medical

DO's

♦ **Adhere to Medication Schedules:** Take all prescribed medicines on time.

♦ **Schedule Regular Check-ups:** Visit your Doctor routinely for health monitoring.

♦ **Conduct Tests Regularly:** Perform necessary medical tests every three to six months as per Doctor advise.

- **Maintain Records:** Keep an organized record of your medical history, illnesses, and treatments.

DO NOT's

- **Hypochondria:** Do not imagine or exaggerate illnesses.

- **Self-Medication:** Avoid self-prescribing medications without consulting a doctor.

- **Avoid Relationships:** Support networks from friends and family are essential for mental health.

6. Support

DO's

- **Seek Help:** Ask for assistance when needed, whether from family, friends, or professionals.

- **Avoid Nagging:** Do not complain excessively to those offering help.

- **Consult Professionals:** Reach out to counsellors or psychiatrists for emotional and psychological support.

- **Hire Caregivers:** Employ a nurse or caregiver if necessary to assist with daily activities.

- **Express Gratitude:** Appreciate and thank those who support you.

- **Avoid Stress:** Strive to minimize stress in your life through relaxation techniques and proper planning.

DO NOT's

- **Overexert:** Resist the urge to manage everything independently.

- **Supress Emotions:** Do not suppress feelings or emotions; talk about them with trusted individuals / friends /near & dear.

- **Feel Like a Burden:** Do not let negative thoughts diminish your sense of self-worth.

Five Daily Habits to be adopted By Seniors around 70's

By the time adults get into their 70s, overall health and well being can vary. Some individuals within this age group are completely healthy, others have multiple health issues, and many fall somewhere in between. Regardless of what's going on health-wise, there are many ways people in their 70s can do every day to maintain Physical, Mental, and Emotional Health. Here are five recommendations to incorporate these in daily routine.

1. **Find Purpose in Life**

   Many of the world's longest-living people report finding purpose in life drives them. This is certainly true for people in their 70 and above. Purpose can involve a variety of meaningful goals and activities, some of which may involve:

- Volunteering in your community.

- Exploring new hobbies like painting, gardening, or writing.

- Sharing stories and experiences with grandchildren or loved ones.

2. Get Sufficient Sleep

It's a myth that older adults need less sleep. In fact, the National Sleep Foundation recommends adults of 65 and above to sleep 7 to 8 hours every night. Chronic health issues and mental health challenges can sometimes affect sleep habits, and your loved one's Doctor should be able to make specific recommendations if such issues are a factor. In general, people in their 70s may enjoy better sleep hygiene by:

- Stick to a consistent bedtime and wake-up schedule.

- Limit excessive daytime naps to maintain night-time sleep quality.

- Stay active during the day to encourage natural fatigue.

- Create a peaceful sleeping environment with minimal noise and proper lighting.

- Avoid drinking too much water before bed to reduce night-time bathroom visits.

3. Avoid Falls

Falls are a significant risk for seniors. The risk of falling becomes greater with each passing decade. One of the ways people in their 70s can minimize this risk is with forms of Yoga exercises that target muscles that play a role in balance and coordination. Gentle forms of exercise such as yoga and water-based activities can help with this goal as well. Reduce this risk by:

- Using anti skid mates, grip bars around toilets and tubs/shower.

- Removing tripping hazards from the home, such as loose rugs or clutter.

- Using Professional Caregivers for additional support if necessary. Elderly home care experts are available to provide high-quality care to seniors on an as-needed basis. From assistance with mobility and exercise to providing transportation to the Doctor's office and social events, there are a variety of ways professional caregivers can help you to continue to live independently.

- Using stool/chair while taking bath.

- Changing clothes in sitting position after coming inside the room only.

4. Keep the Brain Engaged

Mental health is just as important as physical health for people in their 70s. In fact, there's plenty of research suggesting aging brains benefit from regular stimulation, which can also reduce cognitive decline and maintain mental alertness. Reading, working puzzles, and learning new things are just some of the many brain-stimulating activities that can help seniors in their 70s maintain good brain health. The most recent development is super brain yoga, which is described in Appendix -1. Initially, you must take help of yoga instructor.

5. **Get Regular Exercise and Eat Healthy Foods**

These are two things that naturally work well together to produce a wide range of physical, mental, and emotional benefits for people in their 70s. Many studies shown healthy eating has numerous benefits for older adults.

Regular exercises and a balanced diet offer numerous benefits:

- **Exercise** helps maintain bone density, joint strength, and mood through endorphin release.
- Forms of exercise like yoga and daily walking can provide an opportunity to clear the mind and relax.

Balanced diets should include:

- Fruits and vegetables.
- Whole grains, beans, and other healthy starches.
- Low-fat dairy products.
- Lean proteins.

One should avoid processed foods and sugary snacks to maintain energy and overall health.